08-BUS-034

The
Breast Cancer
Survival Manual

The

BREAST
CANCER

·SURVIVAL MANUAL·

A Step-by-Step Guide for Women
with Newly Diagnosed Breast Cancer

SIXTH EDITION

JOHN S. LINK, M.D.,

WITH

SHLOMIT EIN-GAL, M.D.,
AND NANCY LINK, R.D.N.

ST. MARTIN'S GRIFFIN · NEW YORK · ⚌

www.stmartins.com

The Library of Congress Cataloging-in-Publication Data is available upon request.

ISBN 978-1-250-14452-2 (trade paperback)
ISBN 978-1-250-18987-5 (ebook)

Our books may be purchased in bulk for promotional, educational, or business use. Please
contact your local bookseller or the Macmillan Corporate and Premium Sales Department
at 1-800-221-7945, extension 5442, or by email at MacmillanSpecialMarkets@macmillan.com.

Originally published by Owl Books, Henry Holt and Company, LLC

First Owl Books Edition: 1998
Second Owl Books Edition: 2000
Third Owl Books Edition: 2003
Fourth Owl Books Edition: 2007
Fifth Owl Books Edition: 2012

First St. Martin's Griffin Edition: November 2017

10 9 8 7 6 5 4 3 2 1

This book is dedicated to all my patients throughout the years.
You have been my best teachers.

Contents

Acknowledgments

The *Breast Cancer Survival Manual* was conceived almost twenty years ago as a teaching guide for women who came to our breast cancer treatment center, Breastlink, with a newly diagnosed breast cancer. We had no idea our "practice manual" would receive such wide acceptance. This is the sixth edition and has required the most revisions to date because of the major advancements over the past several years.

One of the most important lessons from this book is that optimal breast cancer care and treatment requires the collaboration of dedicated breast specialists working together for *you*. At Breastlink, I have had the privilege of working with leading and outstanding breast cancer treatment teams in Southern California. We have five centers in Southern California and a newly opened center in New York City. Our patients are so fortunate to have talented and dedicated breast surgeons, Drs. John West, Amy Bremner, Lisa Guerra, Lisa Curcio, Hang Dang, and Nimi Kapoor in SoCal and Sharon Rosenbaum Smith, Paul Tartter, and Alison Estabrook in New York City.

The accurate diagnosis and workup of a breast cancer requires excellence in imaging and pathology. We have a superb team of breast imagers that have all done breast specialty fellowships: Drs. June Chen,

Samantha Kubaska, Azita Berashi, Chris Hsu, and Tchaiko Parris. I would like to acknowledge Dr. Shu Yuan Liao and her team at O.C. Pathology for their superb contribution to our patient care.

We work with outstanding radiation oncologists throughout Southern California. I would especially like to thank Drs. Ernie Ngo and Chu Pei Feng for their instrumental role in our IORT program. We are fortunate to have highly skilled plastic/reconstructive breast surgeons at Breastlink, Drs. Justin West and Mark Gaon.

I rely tremendously on my medical oncology colleagues Wade Smith and Shlomit Ein-Gal, who are brilliant and dedicated to delivering the most current treatment possible.

We, the doctors, could not possibly provide the care we do without our dedicated staffs from our front desk receptionists to our medical assistants, our nurse practitioners, physician assistants, and the dozens of staff members that interact with our patients to achieve the best care possible. Research is critical to what we do, and we have a terrific research team under the leadership of Kristi Maya. We have a strong patient support program with survivor volunteers under the direction of Jill Canales and a psychotherapy program under the direction of Lisa Donely.

I would especially like to acknowledge and thank my wife, Nancy Link, R.D.N., who is our nutritional counselor and my coauthor, best critic, supporter, and editor. This edition of *The Breast Cancer Survival Manual* would not have been possible without her tireless effort.

I cannot bypass this opportunity to express gratitude to my parents, who raised me with love and gave me every opportunity to pursue my dreams. Both died far too early from this disease called cancer. My mother provided me with a wonderful New Zealand heritage and taught me to the last days of her life about hope and dignity. My father, a kind and gentle elementary schoolteacher, provided me with a brilliant example of how to live one's life with compassion and grace.

Heroes are a good thing to have and call upon for inspiration. I have had a number of them, but two stand out: my track coach at the University of Southern California, Willie Wilson, who died from cancer when I was nineteen years old, and my boyhood hero, Sir Edmund Hilary. Both of these gentlemen were the epitome of courage and dedication.

Breastlink would not be possible as it is today without the vision and support of Howard Berger, M.D. Dr. Berger, the founder of RAD-NET, took Breastlink ten years ago from a fledgling practice to a bicoastal group of centers that provide state of the art breast cancer treatment and research.

Last, and most important, I would like to thank my patients through the years, as they have been my greatest teachers and are responsible for this book.

—JSL

Introduction

This book is a crisis manual for women who are newly diagnosed with breast cancer. It is the sixth edition of *The Breast Cancer Survival Manual*, which I have written over the past twenty years. The really good news is that the vast majority of women who read this edition of the *Survival Manual* will be cured of breast cancer! This outcome is much more likely than it was twenty years ago because of early diagnosis and new, more effective, and less toxic treatments.

However, breast cancer is still a crisis, and this manual is an attempt to put into words what we do on a daily basis, which is help women who are newly diagnosed with breast cancer understand what they are up against and develop a plan to overcome this obstacle—and, I would even say, achieve a cure.

When women receive the life-threatening and life-altering diagnosis of breast cancer, we ask them to become educated immediately so that they can make critical treatment decisions. We ask this at a time when most are experiencing fear, panic, and disbelief. Regardless of your prior knowledge about the disease or your age or life situation, no one is immune to a natural sense of urgency and fear.

Women probably experience a sense of urgency because they have a perception of breast cancer that is out-of-date: before the 1970s, the one-stage mastectomy, or removal of the entire breast including muscles and lymph nodes (a radical mastectomy), was the only option. With the discovery of a breast lump, surgeons had their patients in the operating room within hours. There was no preoperative workup in those days. If a woman awoke with pain and heavy bandages, she knew it was cancer.

Significant progress has been made since that time. Breast cancer can present as a lump, but more often it presents as an abnormal mammogram before any lump can be felt or noticed. The diagnosis is made by a needle biopsy. Cells are pulled out of the breast and analyzed. If the diagnosis is cancer, there is time—yes, time—to become knowledgeable and prepared, to request second opinions and develop a treatment plan, and to gather together your treatment team.

We have come a long way from the one-step, one-size-fits-all mastectomy. Today every woman's situation is unique, based on how the cancer looks under the microscope, the size of the tumor, and whether cancer cells have spread to the lymph nodes. We are even beginning to look at the mutations in the DNA of the cancer cells. And then there is the woman herself—her age, health, and life situation. Often, surgery is not the first step. Genetic testing may be used to help assess future risks and guide decisions about different treatment options. Chemotherapy or hormone therapy may be used to shrink the tumor before undergoing surgery. The goal of individualized treatment strategies is to achieve a cure with the least amount of side effects. It is important to develop a treatment plan that does not burn any bridges that would be difficult to repair in the future, eliminating other courses of action that could be employed later.

When I say that you have time, I know you are thinking, How much time? I usually tell patients that they have many weeks to learn about their specific disease and develop an individualized treatment plan. You will learn in chapter 1 that the cancer has probably been in your body for several years by the time of diagnosis and that days or weeks are not critical to its development. The important thing is to choose the correct treatments for local and systemic management and decide how the therapies will be sequenced.

I have been helping women plan and manage their breast care for over thirty years. When it became clear that the treatment of breast cancer involved a number of different specialties working together, my dream was to create a center where all breast-dedicated specialists could come together with a single focus: to cure women who have breast cancer. And so this dream became reality twenty-two years ago, when Breastlink was born. There are now a number of Breastlink centers in Southern California and one in New York City.

The old method of treating breast cancer patients is what I call the *sequential* method. A woman with cancer would see a succession of independent doctors, usually beginning with the surgeon, most often a general surgeon. Each physician does what she or he is trained to do but without coordinating with the rest of the medical team. The surgeon operates, the radiation oncologist provides radiation treatment, and the medical oncologist administers chemotherapy. This sequential approach is not well coordinated. In fact, it is common for the physicians to have minimal communication with each other. The optimal approach is *collaborative*, with multiple breast cancer specialists working together to achieve the best outcome for each woman.

Since the first edition of *The Breast Cancer Survival Manual* came out twenty years ago, 90 percent of the information regarding diagnosis and treatment has changed. One of my concerns for recently diagnosed women is that they may consult a physician who does not specialize in breast cancer or who works alone and does not stay completely current with the rapid advancements in research and discoveries that will most benefit breast cancer patients. This is why, even if you are feeling tremendous urgency to start treatment, it is a good idea to take time to become educated and to consider obtaining a comprehensive second opinion. And it is why I have felt compelled to update the manual regularly, now publishing this sixth edition with the latest research incorporated.

At Breastlink centers, we are fortunate to have physician specialists who are dedicated to treating women with breast cancer. Once a breast cancer has been diagnosed and we have collected all the necessary images and pathologic results from the biopsies, our team meets to discuss each woman's unique situation and to develop the appropriate treatment plan. Each of our Breastlink centers has a weekly meeting with all the team members, including the breast radiologist, pathologist, breast surgeon, plastic surgeon, radiation oncologist, medical oncologist, and social worker, as well as members of the clinical research and genetics teams.

New patient cases are presented to the Breastlink treatment team at these weekly meetings, and a thorough discussion leads to development of the individualized treatment plan. In addition, eligibility for research protocols is evaluated. The individual plan is then presented to the patient and her personal support team by the surgeon or oncologist or both. The discussion can be recorded so that we can go back and review it at a later date, if desired. We go over treatment options, the sequencing of treatments, and timelines. At this point a patient may want to take our recommendations to an outside institution or medical group for confirmation or a second opinion, which is something that we completely support.

A woman's case may be presented to the treatment planning conference a second time once surgery is completed or a course of hormonal or chemotherapy has been given. The plan may be modified based on new developments.

It would be a tremendous mistake to treat a breast cancer case without considering the woman herself. A woman's age, hormone status, general health, emotional support, sexuality, immune system, and psychological and spiritual well-being are all extremely important in planning her treatment. Because traditional medicine often neglects treating the whole person, many women seek complementary therapy outside mainstream medicine. At Breastlink, we support a woman's desire to search for comprehensive care and help wherever we can, often with referrals for psychotherapy, physical therapy, yoga, or existential therapy (mindfulness). Our centers also provide access to nutrition counseling and maintain active volunteer and support groups.

We believe complementary care is helpful and supportive to the work we do. Our main task, however, is to cure cancer with the best scientifically proven methods available. In recent years, the field has gotten much more complicated—and also exciting. New discoveries about the human genome allow us to identify mutations that are responsible for and influence cancer. There are more tests, more drugs, and more clinical trials under way than ever before. This book is not designed to teach everything that is known about breast cancer; rather, it is a manual for patients that provides a framework for where we are today and what is likely to come in the future.

In chapter 1, we begin the book with basic information about breast cancer. What is the difference between a normal cell and a cancer cell? We will show you the anatomy of the breast and the microstructures where the first cell mutates. Once a cell mutates and becomes cancerous, it can remain contained in the milk duct—what we call *in situ*—or become invasive and spread beyond the milk duct. We will also discuss growth rates and how cancer spreads into the lymphatic system and blood.

With the basics clarified, in chapter 2 we help you begin your journey. We call this chapter "The Launching Pad." My plan is to help you understand the nature and biology of your specific cancer and how to obtain optimal care. In today's world, where knowledge is power, you will have the confidence to find the right treatment team and, in partnership with them, make the best treatment decisions for you. You will learn how to find the best treatment team, gather and track your records, and obtain a second opinion. We will also explore the current health care systems and how best to navigate them.

Chapter 3 explains the new genomic classification of invasive breast cancer and will allow you to understand your breast cancer type. This is critical because modern treatment is based on the genomic type of your cancer. Chapter 4 helps you understand the pathology reports of your biopsy and breast surgery. This chapter will further help you understand which cancer subtype you fall into: Luminal A, Luminal B, HER2-positive, or triple-negative.

Chapters 5 and 6 are overviews of the two main breast cancer treatment paths: local control (surgery and radiation) and systemic control. I also discuss the sequencing of the treatments because there has been a trend in recent years toward providing systemic therapy before undertaking local control. In the chapter on local control, we discuss the role of reconstructive surgery for patients receiving both mastectomy and partial mastectomy, which we refer to as *wide local excision* (WLE).

Chapter 7 is devoted to the earliest form of breast cancer, *ductal carcinoma in situ* (DCIS). This preinvasive breast cancer accounts for about 20 percent of newly diagnosed cases. It is managed with local control, and the cure rate approaches 100 percent. If you have this early form of breast cancer, you can avoid the chapters on the treatment of invasive breast cancer.

The next three chapters are devoted to the treatment of the invasive breast cancers. Chapter 8 concerns treatment of the hormone-positive Luminal breast cancers. Chapter 9 covers treatment of the HER2-positive type, and chapter 10 discusses the triple-negative type. This is a departure from the last edition of this manual because therapies are now more specifically directed at each subtype based on emerging scientific discoveries and clinical research. When we utilize a more tailored approach, we can avoid unnecessary treatments and use new, less toxic options.

Chapter 11 deals with the genetic predisposition of developing breast cancer. Approximately 10 percent of women inherit a gene from their mother or father that greatly increases the risk of breast cancer. This chapter will help you understand if you might fall into this group and if you should have genetic testing. Since the last edition, multiple genes have been discovered that convey increased risk. This is important for treatment planning, and there are new drugs that specifically target women who have a genetically related breast cancer.

Chapter 12 is about nutrition and healthy lifestyle. We will talk about the concept of *prehabilitation* in preparation for treatment, as well as dietary supplements and proper nutrition during treatment and after. You will almost certainly be inundated with information and recommendations from well-meaning sources about what to eat and which supplements to take, especially if you search the Internet or attend support groups. This chapter will help you put all of that advice into perspective.

Chapter 13 is about breast cancer research and the clinical trial process. It may help you determine if you are eligible and interested in participating in a research trial. Chapter 14 is about life after breast cancer and becoming a survivor. It will help you create an ongoing health care plan based on this new development in your life.

It is our hope that this manual will be helpful to you during a difficult period. Over the past twenty years, our medical practice has been devoted to women with breast cancer, and we have seen the positive effects of patient participation in forming treatment plans. Since more and more physicians today are asking for their patients' input on important decisions regarding treatment, having proper preparation will empower you to become an informed participant in the decision-making process, which is invaluable, given that most women fear their recommended therapy could be inadequate.

Of equal concern, however, is overtreatment. Many women are being overtreated without understanding the true risks, benefits, and appropriateness of the therapy they receive. We hope to alleviate the fear of under- or overtreatment by clearly describing all the options available to you, which you can discuss with your doctors, and by directing you to informational resources.

The main objective of this book is to educate you about breast cancer and to give you some control over what may now seem like chaos. Information is critical and constantly changing. You have access to the latest information on breast cancer diagnosis and treatment through numerous resources, including your medical team, support groups, a wide variety of printed material, and the Internet; see the Resources section at the back of the book for a number of important websites.

Although we have updated the information contained in this manual on a continuing basis (now in our sixth edition), the process stops at the time of publication. To provide you with the latest in breast cancer research, diagnosis, and treatment, we invite you to visit us at http://www.breastlink.com.

We recommend that you use this manual as your breast cancer treatment workbook. Keep notes and highlight important information. As we describe in chapter 2, you may want to begin tracking your personal health history by collecting and managing copies of your medical records. This can be accomplished using a three-ring binder or your computer. There are several personal health record apps available on the Internet, and you can select the one best for you.

Whether you skim *The Breast Cancer Survival Manual* once or it never leaves your side throughout treatment, we hope it will inform and empower you, helping you receive the breast cancer treatment and care that is *right for you* during this challenging time in your life.

Breast Cancer Basics

can•cer *noun* \'kan(t)- sər\ **:** a malignant tumor of potentially un-limited growth that expands locally by invasion and systemically by metastasis

Before beginning our discussion about cancer of the breast, I want to give you some very basic information about cancer in general and how its unique characteristics compare to a normal cell.

Normal body cells can do the following:

- Reproduce themselves EXACTLY.
- Stop reproducing at the right moment.
- Stick together in the correct place.
- Self-destruct if a mistake occurs or they are damaged.
- Mature and become specialized.
- Die (they are programmed to do so) and, when appropriate, they are renewed by *like* cells.

Cancer cells are different from normal cells in the following ways:

- Cancer cells don't stop reproducing.
- Cancer cells don't obey signals from other cells.
- Cancer cells don't stick together; they can break off and float away.
- Cancer cells stay immature and don't specialize, so they become more and more primitive, and they reproduce quickly and haphazardly.
- Cancer cells lose their programmed death pathway.

In this chapter we are going to explore the nature of breast cancer. It is a mystery to us why the female breast is vulnerable to developing cancer. It may have something to do with monthly cycling of glandular cells, yet more than half of breast cancers develop in older women after the breast glands have come to rest. We know that cancer tends to occur in organs with cells that are constantly cycling through cell renewal. The replacement of a cell requires the production of a new set of genes, and this process can lead to mistakes (*mutations*) that the cell is unable to repair. The mistakes can then be repeated, causing a cell to grow according to a new blueprint in a process that is out of control, and this process results in cancer.

First, let's examine the anatomy of the female breast (Figure 1.1). The female breast is composed of milk-producing *lobules* connected to milk *ducts* that carry milk from the lobule to the nipple. There are at least twelve or more of these separate branching ductal-lobular units that occupy the four quadrants of the breast. Supporting and surrounding the glandular units are fibrous tissue, fat cells, blood vessels, and the lymphatic system that drains from the breast to the lymph nodes. We believe that the majority of breast cancers are due to a genetic mistake within the cells lining the *lobules* or *ducts*. There is evidence that genetic mistakes are common, and the majority are harmless. Cells actually have the ability to self-repair these genetic mistakes so that they do not go on to become cancer.

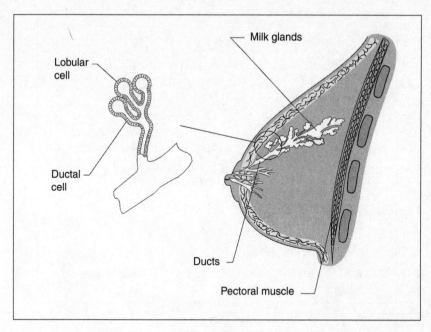

Lobular cell

Ductal cell

Milk glands

Ducts

Pectoral muscle

Figure 1.1
Breast anatomy

A cancer is born when a mistake occurs at a critical point in the cell's genetic blueprint, or *DNA*, and it goes unrepaired. This genetic mistake affects the behavior and characteristics of the affected cell and the new cells that are produced. When a cell becomes genetically un-stable, it has gone bad. These unstable cells continue to divide, pass-ing along the damaged or mutant genetic message to the next generation of cells.

As the new cluster of cancer cells emerges from a milk duct or lob-ule in the breast, it can remain within the duct system (*in situ*), or it can invade the basement membrane and spread into the fat and sup-porting tissue (*invasive* or *infiltrating*). (See Figure 1.2.) This ability to grow and invade is a characteristic of cancer, and it can spread locally, within the breast, or spread into lymph and blood vessels.

The resulting group of cancerous cells (*clone*) can have most of the same characteristics as the normal breast duct cell (i.e., hormone

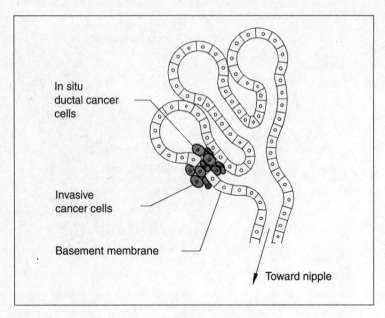

In situ
ductal cancer
cells

Invasive
cancer cells

Basement membrane

Toward nipple

Figure 1.2

In situ and invasive breast cancer

receptors) and grow slowly but steadily. On the other hand, the mutation(s) can lead to a clone that is highly malignant, with the resulting cells having no resemblance to the normal breast cells. We are beginning to understand that not all breast cancers are alike; they behave differently depending on the type of mutation and the resulting proteins or lack of proteins that direct the cell's behavior. We now have the ability to analyze genetic material within cancer cells and map the unique patterns. From this research a new method of classifying breast cancer has emerged (see the discussion in chapter 3).

Breast cancers can remain contained within the duct system (in situ) for months or even years. Some cancers may require an additional mistake (mutation) to invade into the surrounding tissue. Other cancers probably immediately invade the surrounding tissue with the initial mutation. Cancers that remain in the duct system are called *ductal carcinoma in situ* (DCIS). (We discuss these preinvasive cancers in chapter 7.) If we can discover a DCIS before it invades the surrounding tissue, there is no risk of its spreading to the body, and the cancer is highly curable with local treatment measures.

The rate of growth of a cancer varies considerably and is very dependent on the mutation that has occurred. Some breast cancers retain the ability to be influenced by hormones (estrogen), and the presence or lack of estrogen will influence their growth.

The genetic blueprint (DNA) within a cancer cell is unstable, and with continued growth further mutations occur. Some of these mutations are so unstable that they become lethal to the cell population itself, thus ending the cancer growth. We tend to think of cancers as "strong" rogue cells. In reality many cancer cells, especially the most malignant, are fragile and just hanging on. Current treatments are able to take advantage of this fragile state and in the future, treatments will target this vulnerability.

As stated earlier, the rate of growth of breast cancer cells varies considerably. The slower growing cancers of the Luminal A type (see chapter 3) take six or more months to double in size (Figure 1.3), while the triple-negative (basal-type) cancers can double in size in weeks to months. The ability to spread into the lymph system and bloodstream depends on the underlying DNA mutation and the size of the cancer. Most cancers cannot spread into lymph and blood vessels (*metastasis*) until they exceed about 1 centimeter (10 mm) in size (see Figure 1.4). We believe that over time slower-growing cancers can further mutate

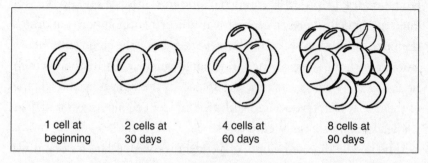

| 1 cell at beginning | 2 cells at 30 days | 4 cells at 60 days | 8 cells at 90 days |

Figure 1.3
Growth of cancer cells over time

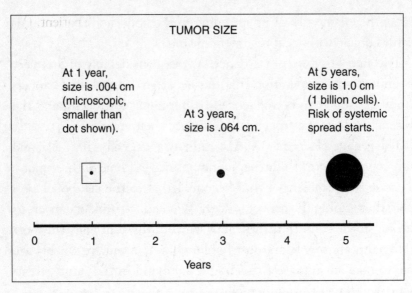

Figure 1.4

Tumor growth over time of a Luminal breast cancer

and increase their growth rate, potential to spread, and degree of malignancy.

Once a cancer has become invasive, there is risk of its spreading into the lymphatic system and the bloodstream. We are not sure what mechanism a cancer cell uses to invade vessels, but it is thought that the process requires DNA programming or mutation. Women often ask if a needle biopsy can disrupt cells and cause them to spread into the lymph nodes. I think this can occur, and in some cases we do see isolated tumor cells shortly after biopsy in the first lymph node that drains the breast. But we also know these women have the same outcome as women without the presence of isolated tumor cells in their lymph nodes. Evidence suggests that the spread to the lymph by the trauma of the biopsy is not associated with true cancer cell metastasis and does not lead to a decrease in cure rates.

The needle-directed biopsy of a cancer is the standard for diagnosis of breast cancer. From this small core of tissue, about the size of a pencil lead, the type of breast cancer can be determined, allowing the treatment team to plan therapy most appropriate for the patient. (We discuss the analysis of tumor tissue more completely in chapter 4.)

In the past we placed huge importance in staging a cancer on analysis of the draining lymph nodes, looking for spread of tumor cells and extent of the spread. Figure 1.5 demonstrates the distribution of lymph nodes draining the breast. Surgeons used to remove a majority of the lymph nodes at the time of the breast cancer surgery. Spread to lymph nodes is an important factor to determine your *prognosis* (probable course or outcome of the disease), but it is no longer necessary to do extensive lymph node surgery. There is increased risk of *lymphedema* (arm swelling) that does not justify the information gained through removal of the majority of nodes. Instead, by removing the *sentinel*

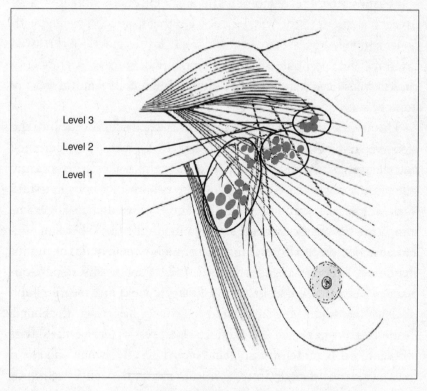

Level 3
Level 2
Level 1

Figure 1.5
Distribution of axillary lymph nodes

node (the first draining lymph node; see chapter 6), we can obtain the needed information without the risks of more extensive surgery. If there is extensive lymph node involvement at the time of diagnosis, the involved lymph nodes are usually treated with systemic therapy, followed by radiation and in some cases surgery.

Historically, lymph node involvement was the strongest predictor of risk of spread into the bloodstream. This is changing. Using a number of tests that can be performed on the needle biopsy, we have greatly improved our ability to assess the risk of cancer spread. (This topic is discussed further in chapters 4 and 6.)

It is important to treat cancer in the lymph nodes draining from the breast. By using sentinel lymph node sampling, ultrasound, and other imaging techniques such as MRI and PET scans, we can plan approaches that use combined therapies for those women whose cancer has spread to the lymph nodes. For the majority of women with no lymph node involvement or microscopic involvement, we can avoid extensive and potentially damaging lymph node surgery. A number of clinical trials have demonstrated that full lymph node removal *does not* improve survival rates.

The most serious and dangerous event is when cells invade into the blood vessels and metastasize into the body. We call this occurrence *systemic spread*. Current technology does not allow us to detect early systemic disease because imaging tests are not sensitive enough to find microscopic cells within the body. A number of researchers are examining ways to detect cancer cells circulating in the blood by using special antibody preparations. This line of inquiry is very promising for the future, although more work needs to be done to ensure development of a test that is consistently accurate, reliable, and meaningful.

Once invasion has occurred and the cancer has grown to about 1 centimeter, it can attract and produce blood vessels (*angiogenesis*) that allow it to break off (*metastasize*) and spread into the lymph and blood system (systemic spread). In this critical process, the cancer cells produce protein messengers known as *vascular endothelial growth factors* (VEGF). To counteract the effects of VEGF, researchers have developed a number of antibodies and molecules that hopefully will be proved to reduce or prevent angiogenesis and ultimately lead to the destruction of the cancer.

With new technologies such as *reverse transcription-polymerase chain reaction* (RT-PCR), researchers are able to compare the genetic blueprint of a normal cell to the transformed malignant cell and identify the abnormal mutant genes. Identification of abnormal gene patterns has led to a new classification (*typing*) system for breast cancer that will be discussed in chapter 3. This ability to analyze the mutant genes has also led to the recognition that some of the abnormalities are related to cancer cell functions such as invasion, proliferation (cell growth), angiogenesis, and metastasis.

Using these techniques, commercial laboratories have been able to analyze cancer cells for the presence of mutant genes associated with systemic spread and to develop tests that can predict how likely a cancer is to recur or metastasize. A number of these *prognostic* (predictors) tests have been developed. They are now available to oncologists to use in making decisions about systemic therapy. With the discovery of over one hundred mutations in breast cancer DNA, tests are being developed that can detect these mutations in DNA fragments that circulate in the blood. This test, called *cell-free DNA*, will allow us to identify cancer mutations without doing a tumor biopsy. It will allow us to select potential targeted treatment options.

Because we can now modify gene mutations, it is possible to develop therapies targeted at the specific mutations; these therapies can reverse the effects of these mutations and potentially reverse the malignant process. In previous editions of this book, I alluded to this possibility, which has now become a reality.

The Launching Pad

KNOWLEDGE IS POWER & SECOND OPINIONS

You may feel frightened and overwhelmed at this point, which is not unusual. When I see a newly diagnosed patient, I tell her that the chance of being cured (yes, cured!) is very high. You do have time to educate yourself, gather information, and even obtain a second opinion if desired. Just remember, take one step at a time! Let me show you how.

The modern diagnosis of breast cancer is made with a needle biopsy following an abnormal mammogram or after a lump is discovered, typically by you, your spouse or partner, or your physician. At this point women often feel a tremendous urgency to have the breast cancer surgically removed RIGHT NOW! It bears repeating: you do have time to gather information and decide on a comprehensive and appropriate treatment plan.

There have been tremendous advancements in our understanding of breast cancer in recent years. We now know that breast cancer is not the same in every woman; it is different, or *heterogeneous*. The more we learn about the nature of breast cancer, the more effective and targeted the therapy we can recommend, and the greater chance you will receive the appropriate care. In most cases optimal treatment planning can be done effectively with comprehensive imaging and needle biopsy prior to embarking on any major surgery.

With modern imaging using mammography, ultrasound, and MRI, we can accurately determine the size and extent of the cancer. Carefully examining the cancer tissue biopsy under the microscope, we can learn a great deal about your specific cancer—that is, the cell type, the different receptors on the cell surface, and how aggressive the malignancy is. (We will explain all of this thoroughly in the next several chapters.) Armed with as much information as we can gather about your cancer, we are able to establish the most effective treatment options.

Interestingly, despite advancements in our understanding of breast cancer, the fundamentals of treatment have not changed significantly over time. We continue to be governed by the concepts of *local control* and *systemic control*. Here is a brief explanation of these two very important concepts in cancer treatment. (Chapters 5 and 6 provide a detailed discussion of this topic.)

- *Local control* is achieved by mapping the location of the cancer in the breast and lymph nodes and then using appropriate and effective treatments to eliminate it before it has had a chance to spread beyond its place of origin.
- If there is a chance that cancer cells have escaped from the original tumor into the rest of the body (the *system*), these cells must also be eliminated in a process referred to as *systemic control*.

Women start this journey in different medical systems. Regardless of the medical system you are in, you are still able to receive coordinated care. The ultimate goal is to survive the cancer with the least amount of side effects and disability.

The United States is currently struggling to reformulate its health care system. As it stands in 2018, women covered by traditional insurance plans have access to physicians and specialists of their own choosing. The alternative system limits patient choices to a group of physicians and specialists who are members of an organized group. You can get excellent care in both types of health care systems, but this will require education, understanding, and oversight on your part. Both systems have advantages and disadvantages.

Traditional Fee-for-Service Health Insurance Model

- A newly diagnosed patient has the freedom to access individual doctors who are in private practice. This allows the patient to seek out potential specialists of her own choosing based on reputation, recommendation, or referral.
- The patient can seek out and select a surgeon or oncologist who specializes primarily in breast cancer.
- Another plus is the patient's access to cutting-edge, outside-the-box treatments.
- One disadvantage of this system is that there is no guarantee that the selected specialists will work together as a treatment team or that they will work within a system of collaborative management. The risk is that decision-making will be made independent of the other treating specialists without development of a comprehensive plan.
- There is also no guarantee that the independent specialists will work together toward a coordinated treatment plan or that one of them will be responsible for performing the job of team leader.

Managed Care Health Insurance Model

- The main potential advantage of a managed care system is that specific guidelines can be put in place, including planning and treatment conferences and established protocols for breast cancer diagnosis and treatment. This can ensure consistency in diagnostic and treatment regimens through standardized procedures.
- Another advantage in some cases is the sharing of electronic med-

ical records databases, which allows all treatment team members to easily follow treatment activities and for ongoing review of the quality of care and analysis of outcomes.

- One disadvantage is that patients are usually locked into the system and cannot go outside it for treatment.
- There is often some restriction on use of cutting-edge drugs or technology until there is absolute scientific evidence to support them from a cost-benefit perspective. In no way does this mean that you cannot get excellent care in this type of system. (In fact, premature use of new technology may not always lead to a better outcome.)
- There may not be access to surgeons or oncologists who specialize exclusively in breast cancer.

Regardless of the system you are in, your understanding of and involvement in your health care are equally important, and you should feel empowered to advocate on your own behalf. This might involve obtaining additional knowledge and education (this manual is a good place to start) or obtaining a second opinion.

Once your cancer diagnosis has been confirmed, by needle biopsy or abnormal mammogram, and the extent of the cancer has been established by breast and lymph node imaging, the next step is to select your treatment team.

Picking the Treatment Team and Coordinating Care

🦋 The diagnosis and treatment of breast cancer have changed dramatically over the past thirty years. Back then a majority of women who had a palpable breast lump went directly into surgery. Often the operation was a mastectomy, and that was the full extent of their treatment. Researchers were just beginning to explore the role of *adjuvant chemotherapy*, and *radiation* was a new kind of treatment utilized by a few brave women.

Today, the majority of breast cancers are discovered by mammography. These cancers are small, often too small to be felt, and surgeons rely on radiologists to find or *localize* them with a hook wire or injected blue dye. As you can see, the technology has changed dramatically, and we have entered a new era of breast cancer diagnosis and therapy. Because of the many elements that come into play in cancer diagnosis and treatment, coordination is critical among a team of physicians: surgeon, radiologist, pathologist, radiation oncologist, plastic surgeon, and medical oncologist.

Ideally, a woman with a newly diagnosed breast cancer connects with a key physician who takes charge of developing a treatment plan with her and who then coordinates the implementation of the plan with the other team members. The group of physicians can work at a single institution or be drawn from a wider geographic area, and any of the cancer specialists can act as the coordinating doctor. At Breastlink, it is usually the medical oncologist who coordinates the flow of information and treatment for a patient, but our surgeons can take on this pivotal role as well. Each patient is presented to our entire group at what we call our pretreatment planning conference (discussed below).

We hope you will find a cancer specialist you can communicate with comfortably and who will address your concerns. However, there are medical systems in which it may be difficult for the patient to connect with one physician who will act as the coordinating team leader. If this describes your situation, don't despair. This manual will give you some information and suggestions to help you function as your own team leader. It is possible to go through this process without a physician to spearhead your treatment plan and still receive state-of-the-art care.

The overall treatment plan revolves around two critical decisions. The first deals with *local control* and the second with the need for *systemic therapy*. Often you and your doctors cannot decide on the issue of systemic therapy until all the information is available from the needle biopsy or from the surgical procedure.

Since the diagnosis and treatment of breast cancer is achieved primarily in an outpatient setting, you may travel to various locations for different aspects of your care. In our community, some women come to our center for surgery and then have radiation at a facility closer to their home. If you require various therapies, you may want to consider coordinating something similar in order to make your treatment appointments as convenient as possible.

From your first decision about whom to contact for your breast cancer care all the way through the many follow-up exams after your treatment is completed, communication is key. Establish a relationship with a physician that will enable you to develop an overall treatment plan that will flow as smoothly as possible. You should also get to know the nurses and other medical staff well. Nurse specialists often play very important roles by coordinating and facilitating the communication process between you and your doctors.

At our Breastlink centers, one of the key tools used in coordinating a woman's care is the pretreatment planning conference. This conference is a meeting of the medical team members to discuss each patient's case and to develop a coordinated treatment plan. The conference allows all team members to review the health history, radiological breast images, pathology report, and pathology slides. In our system, the patient does not participate in the treatment planning conference. After the conference, you should be apprised of the process and the conclusions reached by the team. Some centers actually give patients formal minutes or written conclusions. Other centers arrange for the conclusions to be verbally presented to you by the team member who is coordinating your care. Usually, the discussion and recommendations made at the pretreatment planning conference are shared with you by the physician who presented your case at the group meeting.

The treatment planning conference is extremely important in coordinating care. Each of the potential treating physicians can, in one setting, agree on an overall treatment plan and his or her particular contribution to that plan. This united approach also guarantees that the doctors line up the sequencing of the different therapies correctly and in the manner that is most beneficial to the overall well-being of the patient. The conference also allows us to identify women who are eligible for special research studies and protocols sponsored by the government or other research groups. At Breastlink this important aspect provides our patients with state-of-the-art care and promotes medical advancement.

Besides benefiting the patient, the nature of the conference promotes education and understanding on the part of the various physicians involved. Younger or new physicians and those in training are often invited to attend the pretreatment planning conference. This is an invaluable experience since they are exposed to a wide variety of patients and situations, which would otherwise take years to accomplish in their own practices. In addition, women diagnosed in the future will benefit greatly from the wealth of knowledge that these conferences provide medical professionals.

Seeking a Second Opinion

❦ Once the treatment team has been selected and a plan developed, many women find it helpful to seek a second opinion so that they have confidence in the diagnosis and treatment plan before commencing with the chosen course of action. It is important for us to note that many women and their families feel anxious or guilty about asking the diagnosing physician to help them gather materials and records to give to another physician or institution for a second opinion. *You don't need to worry about this.* It has become such a common practice that physicians are neither surprised nor insulted by such requests.

There are several important reasons to get a second opinion when you have been diagnosed with breast cancer. Even when you trust your physicians completely, the gravity of a cancer diagnosis demands that you feel fully confident with the diagnosis and treatment plan before proceeding any further. A second opinion that concurs with the first opinion can give you that confidence. Although confirmation is reassuring, a second opinion can also add to or conflict with information you have already received. Remember that both *conflicting* and *confirming* data will help establish productive dialogue that can lead to a more appropriate treatment plan and a better understanding of your unique situation.

You might think that breast cancer is so common that the recommended treatment must be fairly standard among doctors. This was more true twenty years ago, when our understanding of breast cancer was much less sophisticated and the treatment options were limited. Current treatment involves a wealth of new tests, *agents* (medicines), and procedures. You want to receive the very best that medicine can offer today, with treatment options tailored specifically for you and your diagnosis.

At Breastlink we diagnose hundreds of women with breast cancer every year. We also render hundreds of second opinions to women with newly diagnosed breast cancer who come to us from other facilities around the United States and around the world. Even though we are regarded as experts in the field, we understand a woman's need to hear confirmation from another source. In any way we can, we encourage and facilitate obtaining a second opinion for any patient. We feel it is extremely important that every woman be comfortable with and have confidence in her treatment team. We welcome outside opinions before embarking on a course of therapy. Occasionally, new information is brought forth from another source, or a different approach is presented that is better suited to the patient. Do not be afraid or hesitant about requesting a second opinion; your doctor should not be concerned about your receiving one. On the contrary, this process is usually encouraged, and any center or physician that discourages a second opinion should be willing to discuss their reasons with you for not supporting this very important issue.

A thorough, comprehensive second opinion takes time and may be expensive—between $500 and $2,000. (Some insurance plans pay for second opinions.) The second opinion should include an independent review of the biopsy tissue by a well-trained pathologist in breast disease, a review of X-rays and imaging studies by a breast radiologist, and presentation to a treatment team for review and recommendations for a treatment plan. This process requires the integration of a team of experienced specialists. The second opinion is usually enlightening, confirming information you already obtained from your diagnosing doctor and from your own independent research.

Occasionally, the second opinion differs drastically from the first, placing you in a dilemma. If the institution rendering the differing opinion is experienced and reputable, the medical team will explain the basis of their opinion to you and your diagnosing physicians. You might ask how, in this age of modern medicine, there can be a major difference in opinion about managing an individual's breast cancer. In our experience, second opinions most often suggest a different sequencing of treatment, caution against overtreatment, or offer alternate medication options.

Breast cancer testing and treatment are constantly evolving, and occasionally physicians may be practicing *older*—out of date—medicine. Newer treatments are often targeted directly at the cancer and are therefore less toxic for the rest of the body. New tools and genetic analysis help us plan appropriate, optimal treatment, but some physicians may not be utilizing all available technologies. Finally, while a mistake in the initial diagnosis is rare, a review of the actual biopsy tissue and of the radiologic images is a must. Sometimes a third opinion is necessary when there is a major difference between your first and second opinions. This should be rendered by a center that specializes in breast cancer treatment. In our practice we sometimes see women who are seeking a fourth or even a fifth opinion. Additional opinions beyond the third will usually differ little and will only delay your decision regarding a treatment plan and the commencement of treatment.

Differences in opinion may affect your medical outcome, or they may be as minor as a different sequencing of therapy (the order in which you receive treatments). A second opinion may propose a different type of chemotherapy, radiation, or hormone therapy, but with a very similar medical outcome to that predicted in the first opinion. Some recommendations may lead to different side effects or affect their duration, experiences that are much less critical and do not affect survival. The point is there may be differences in opinion, and some are minor and some are major.

Frequently encountered differences in opinion

1. Extent of breast surgery—mastectomy versus *partial mastectomy* (breast conservation)
2. Extent of lymph node sampling
3. Need for radiation combined with surgery
4. The type of radiation
5. The need for and type of systemic treatment
6. Sequencing of systemic treatment and surgery
7. Eligibility for a research protocol

There may also be differences regarding radiation therapy, chemotherapy, or hormonal therapy. The type and intensity of the therapy recommended may differ depending on the experience and judgment of the physicians involved. Recommendations may also differ if a new technology or research protocol is uniquely available at an institution. Research protocols that have unproven benefit and carry risk to the patient need to be thoroughly explained and require an informed consent. Just because it's new doesn't mean it's better! *New* becomes better only after scientific confirmation, followed by government review and approval as a standard therapy. Women diagnosed with breast cancer certainly can consider participating in a clinical trial if appropriate and available (the focus of chapter 13).

You should start the process of obtaining a second opinion as soon as possible after you make the decision to seek one. Your diagnosing doctor may be helpful in recommending a physician or facility that specializes in breast cancer treatment, such as a university, a large urban hospital, or a private facility. The process of securing another doctor's or team's opinion involves several steps and may take a week or more to complete. We believe the best second opinion for women with newly diagnosed breast cancer is multidisciplinary and requires a thorough review of imaging and pathology, so be sure you provide complete documentation from your diagnosis.

The following items will be needed:

Copies of all breast imaging, including mammograms, ultrasounds, and MRIs (if an image-guided biopsy was performed, include the images of the breast biopsy and postbiopsy)
Pathology slides and reports
Results from blood work
Body scans (if applicable)

These items can be collected by you for delivery in person or shipped by an overnight carrier, which will track and guarantee delivery. Electronic documents, images, and scans can also be emailed directly from you or from your diagnosing doctor's office. In addition, most facilities will give you a health-history questionnaire that includes space for you to provide a thorough family history of breast cancer on your mother's and father's sides of the family. The second-opinion coordinator will most likely send or email you this questionnaire, to be completed and returned by email or in person at the time of the consult.

It is not always necessary to obtain a second opinion in person. Traditionally, patients seeking additional expert advice would schedule an appointment with a local physician or medical center; take along to this appointment the pathology report, biopsy slides, and imaging pictures from their diagnosing doctors; and obtain an in-person second opinion. Now you can have your images and pathology and any pertinent records reviewed and then have a live "telemedicine" interaction with the expert on your smartphone or computer. At Breastlink, we have such a service, called TeleLink. You can learn more about this service at www.breastlink.com. If you desire a second opinion from someone whom you consider to be a breast cancer expert, whether that person is in your state, somewhere else in the United States, or even in another country, this can be accomplished. The second opinion can be delivered to you electronically or by regular mail so that you can review it and discuss the recommendations with your treating physician.

Based on your medical records, images, and pathology, the second opinion specialist(s) will present their assessment of your diagnosis, recommend treatment options, and discuss the risks and benefits of those options. The price you pay for this time and expertise will be money well spent. You should feel confident your diagnosis is correct and be comfortable with the information you have received. Remember, differences in approach and treatment do occur. What is extremely important in a second opinion is to confirm the cancer diagnosis and the results from the pathology so that you receive the appropriate treatment for your type and extent of cancer. A misdiagnosis in this area can lead to over- or undertreatment; a second opinion can help reduce either possibility.

For the most part, physicians, like people everywhere, have different ways of approaching a problem, believe that what they are doing is best, and have reasons for their treatment choices. You must consider the opinions presented and choose the treatment plan that is right for you. There is a good chance that the second opinion will simply confirm the diagnosis and treatment suggested by your first doctor.

Armed with your first and second opinions and the reading and research you have done, you are now ready to review all the information with your physician and settle on a comprehensive treatment plan. This may be hard for you to believe, but you can reach this point in two to three weeks. While you may think you are not capable enough or comfortable enough to be involved in this decision process you may be pleasantly surprised. Most physicians want their patients to be well-informed, active participants. In the upcoming weeks, you will find that your confidence and desire to participate in your own care will increase with the amount of information and guidance you have. It is not a path you would have chosen, but it is one you must take, and the better prepared you are, the safer the journey!

To help you compare the information provided in first and second opinions, we have included the accompanying worksheet (worksheet 2.1).

Working Within the Medical System

✂ Medical offices all function and work differently. It would be ideal to have access to every doctor in every office whenever you need them, but this is not always possible. The following are a few key points to help you navigate the different medical systems.

- Carry a notebook or electronic record-keeping tool that is set up to record information received from the different medical offices.
- Have at hand all necessary contact information, including names and telephone numbers.
- Discuss how best to communicate with your medical team: telephone, email, etc.
- Ask about the procedures for urgent assistance. (Your own doctor may not be available, but that is okay. You will speak either to the doctor on call or to other medical personnel responsible for helping you.)
- Inquire at each medical office how you can obtain a copy of your personal records.
- Learn the name and telephone number of the person at every office who is responsible for the business aspects of your treatment, who processes insurance claims, treatment authorizations, requests for medical records, etc.

There is nothing more distressing than being diagnosed with cancer and then having to deal in a new environment that is intimidating and foreign at the same time. Many find this combination simply

SECOND OPINION WORKSHEET			
Tumor Characteristics and Opinions			Notes and Decisions
	Primary Opinion	Second Opinion	
SIZE			
Palpable			
Mammogram			
Ultrasound			
PATHOLOGY			
Invasive			
Noninvasive			
Histologic grade			
Hormone +/–			
HER2 +/–			
Lymph nodes			
TREATMENT			
Local control			
Systemic control			
FOLLOW-UP			
Hormonal			
Surveillance			
Clinical trials			

Worksheet 2.1

Second opinion worksheet

overwhelming. Your task is further complicated by the fact that you will need to see a number of different physician specialists, requiring you to interact and coordinate several different offices and treatment facilities at the same time.

Every office and treatment facility has key individuals you will get to know. There is usually a clinical person (registered nurse, nurse practitioner, or physician's assistant) who works closely with the physician, and whom you can contact between office visits for any questions or concerns. This person has direct access to your doctor and can act as your advocate, especially if he or she knows you and is familiar with your current medical and treatment status. The nurse or nurse practitioner can most likely get to the physician faster than you can, so for this reason we recommend that you utilize this team member as your first choice for help. To address key specific issues with your doctor, be sure to keep a list of your concerns and questions so that you don't forget anything at your next office visit. In the next section we will discuss the importance of collecting and managing your personal health records.

Your Medical Information and Experiences

Maintain Your Medical Records

We believe it is important for all patients to track their personal health information. By keeping up-to-date, easily accessible health records you will play an active role in your breast cancer treatment and become an informed and knowledgeable participant in your care and survival plan. Maintaining your breast cancer medical records will help you to

- keep track of every aspect of your care,
- provide easy and direct access to your complete breast cancer medical history,
- know and understand your personal breast cancer diagnosis and treatment plan,

- easily retain and share medical information with health care providers,
- ensure that all members of your medical team are informed and united on the course of your care,
- avoid the possibility of incorrect treatment,
- reduce or eliminate the potential for duplicate procedures or tests,
- prevent delays in treatment and decision-making.

We suggest you adopt an organized approach to collecting your medical information right from the start. You can collect, organize, and store your medical information in a number of different ways:

1. Simply gather your paper records and file them in a three-ring binder using tabs for the various types of documents (e.g., physician or medical office contact information, insurance records, office visit notes, pathology reports, surgical procedures, chemotherapy treatment schedule, appointment calendar, and so on).

2. Create a folder in your personal computer and transfer medical records obtained electronically from your health care providers into the dedicated location. You can sort your medical documents into different subfolders within your breast cancer folder, such as those described above.

3. Subscribe to a Web-based app that allows you to enter and access your health information by computer at any time. Using a Web-based medical records app allows you to receive and store all personal health documents related to your breast cancer diagnosis and treatment, including radiology images, surgical reports, lab results, chemotherapy regimen, appointment calendar, office visit notes, pharmacy and prescription records, and much more.

Whichever method you use will allow you to retain a complete picture of your breast cancer history that you can review at any time and, if you choose, to share with family, friends, or other health care providers. Your health information will most likely be scattered across many different medical facilities and provider offices, so you will want to establish how these individual sites will provide information to you, whether by paper copy, email, or through another type of electronic transmission such as fax or e-fax. Having direct access to your medical records allows you the opportunity and ability to absorb complex information about your diagnosis, treatment, and test results and to actively participate in your survival.

Record Medical Sessions

At our breast care centers, we routinely record consultations and second opinion sessions. The best way to do this is on your cell phone, which is easy and convenient. We understand that an extensive amount of information is exchanged that may be new to you or that you might not remember due to feelings of anxiety, stress, or fear. If a member of your personal support team cannot attend the consultation with you, then obtaining a recording of the session will provide you with an accurate accounting to share later. Through review of the recorded session you will have an opportunity to more fully absorb the information presented and many of your questions may be answered.

Keep a Personal Journal

The process of writing down your experiences, thoughts, and feelings can be very beneficial and healing. Researchers at the University of Texas at Austin and North Dakota State University examined healthy people and found that those who write in journals about their deepest thoughts and feelings of difficult events have stronger immunity than those who don't. Another group of researchers from the State University of New York at Stonybrook showed that writing about a stressful experience reduces physical symptoms in patients with chronic illness. Journal writing provides you with the gentlest and safest of therapies. No expertise is required and it is a great way to express yourself without fear of consequence.

Get the Most from Your Appointments

We want your experience at the doctor's office to be as productive as possible. At your initial appointment, you will get details about your breast cancer diagnosis and your treatment options. It's a good idea to bring a list of questions for the doctor. As noted earlier, you might ask if you can record the sessions if no recordings will be provided. You should consider bringing a loved one or a close friend along with you to help you gather and retain information as well as to provide comfort and reassurance.

The next step is to proceed through the following chapters to ensure that you have a basic knowledge of your breast cancer. By developing a good understanding, you will be sure to ask the questions that are most important in making a truly informed decision. And remember: just take it one step at a time!

3

......

❧

Types of Breast Cancer

Over the last several years there has been tremendous scientific progress in understanding the different gene mutations found in breast cancers. As a result, a classification system for naming breast cancer has emerged. In the past, breast cancer was classified by several different characteristics: (1) the type of cell where the tumor originated (ductal vs. lobular), (2) how different the cancer cell was from the normal breast cell (*differentiation*), and (3) whether the cancer cell contained unique receptors on its surface.

The classification now being used by research scientists and the medical community was established using a gene-analysis technique called *microarray analysis*. In this method of analysis, breast cancer cells are very closely examined (*sequenced*) in the laboratory using special equipment. The results of this analysis have identified four distinct breast cancer types:

1. Luminal A
2. Luminal B
3. Basal cell (also called triple-negative)
4. HER2-positive

Each type presents a different pattern of growth, different ability to spread beyond the breast, and different disease outcome. Establishing your breast cancer type will help guide your medical team to the best treatment options for you.

Until several years ago, an individual woman's tumor tissue did not routinely undergo microarray analysis since the technique is expensive and was generally used as a research tool. However, specialty laboratories now offer commercially available microarray analysis to identify the four different breast cancer types. Even without microarray analysis, your cancer will still be categorized into one of the four types based on the following: (1) the way it looks under the microscope (the unique characteristics of the cancer cell and how much it looks like or differs in appearance from a normal cell), (2) where the cancer began (duct or lobule), (3) the presence or absence of hormone receptors (estrogen and progesterone) on the surface of the cancer cell, and (4) the production of a cancer gene known as the *HER2 oncogene*.

The incidence of each of the four breast cancer types is presented in the accompanying pie graph (Figure 3.1). Your pathology report may not list your type, but this practice is changing, and in the future typing information will be included routinely on pathology reports.

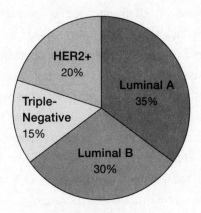

Figure 3.1
Distribution of breast cancer types

Using the descriptions that follow, you can easily determine your type, and your oncologist will certainly work with you to understand which category your tumor falls into. Chapters 8, 9, and 10 describe the treatment regimens appropriate for each of these breast cancer types.

Luminal A Breast Cancer

Luminal A cancers are slow-growing, *low-grade* cancers. They are the breast cancers most frequently discovered by screening mammograms. In the older classification, the Luminal A cancers were the well-differentiated (meaning the cancer cells closely resemble normal cells), grade 1 (or low-grade) ductal cancers (originating in the milk duct). These low-grade breast cancers have excellent outcomes, with cure rates in excess of 90 percent. Subtypes of Luminal A cancers include tubular, papillary, cribriform, and mucinous (also known as colloid) cancers; this terminology is used to describe how the cancer cells appear under the microscope. All Luminal A cancers are estrogen- and progesterone-positive, which means that they have both estrogen and progesterone receptors on the cancer cell surface. They are considered low-grade based on their *modified Bloom-Richardson score* (see chapter 4), and they lack the HER2 overproduction.

When specialized testing is conducted on Luminal A cancer cells, they are found to be very similar to a normal breast tissue cell. The more a cancer cell looks like a normal cell, the more it will behave like one. For this reason I believe we must be careful not to overtreat this cancer type. Luminal A cancers tend to develop in a single site in the breast (*unifocal*) and to remain in that place without spreading into the lymph system or bloodstream. These cancers can be cured with limited surgery and radiation and do not require chemotherapy.

One of the current controversies about Luminal A breast cancers is whether this type can further mutate and change its DNA blueprint over time to become a Luminal B cancer; certain scientific evidence suggests that this can occur. Pathologists examining Luminal A tumor tissue under the microscope sometimes observe an area within the cancer that appears to be different and has a higher *proliferative rate* (growth rate). If left to continue growing, this mutated group of cells (called a *clone*) can overtake the surrounding slower-growing Luminal A cancer cells. As further evidence, we rarely find a grade 1 cancer larger than 2 centimeters. It is thought that before the Luminal A cancer reaches 2 centimeters it changes into the more aggressive Luminal B type. I believe this is why screening and early diagnosis are so important, in order to find small cancers before they have a chance to change and become more dangerous.

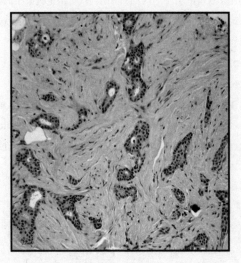

Figure 3.2
Luminal A breast cancer

Luminal B Breast Cancer

✘ In the old classification, Luminal B cancers were termed intermediate-grade ductal cancers, or infiltrating lobular cancers. Sometimes they are a mixture of both ductal and infiltrating lobular cancers, which is called *mammary carcinoma*. As stated in the previous section, some Luminal A cancers probably become Luminal B over time. These transformed cancers tend to be more aggressive in their growth and spread than Luminal A. They are estrogen-receptor-positive but often lose the progesterone receptor from the cancer cell surface. They do not overproduce the HER2 oncogene. Luminal B cancers have a higher proliferative rate (growth rate) and increased *Ki67 score* (a measure of how quickly cancer cells are growing) than Luminal A cancers.

Cancers with a *lobular* pattern are frequently *multifocal* (the cancer develops at multiple sites within one quadrant of the breast) and have *skipped* areas of normal breast tissue in between. The mammogram will often underestimate the size of the primary cancer and not identify the secondary *satellite* cancers. For this reason, MRI is often a very helpful imaging tool with Luminal B cancers.

Treatment of Luminal B cancers requires special considerations. Local control requires removing the cancer completely from the breast, and because of the multifocality and difficulty determining the extent of the cancer on physical exam and imaging, complete removal is often challenging. It is not unusual to find cancer at the edge of the

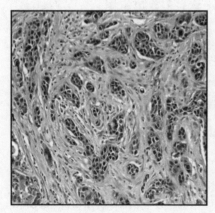

Figure 3.3a

Luminal B: ductal subtype

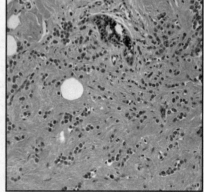

Figure 3.3b

Luminal B: lobular subtype

removed breast tissue (*positive margins*), making a second surgery necessary to achieve *clear margins*. Compared with Luminal A cancers, Luminal B cancers have a greater ability or propensity to spread through the lymph and blood vessels. New technologies using *gene profiling* have helped the medical oncologist determine those women who will benefit from chemotherapy after surgery. (Treatment for Luminal B cancers is discussed further in chapter 8.)

Basal-Type or Triple-Negative

✂ Basal-type cancers account for about 15 percent of all breast cancer. These cancers are also termed *triple-negative* (the term most frequently used by the medical and patient community) because they often lack both estrogen and progesterone hormone receptors on their cell surfaces and they do not overproduce the HER2 oncogene. Close to 90 percent of basal-type cancers are truly triple-negative. The remaining 10 percent do have some degree of hormone positivity on the cell surface but do not respond to hormone therapy.

Triple-negative cancers are very proliferative, with high Ki67 percentage and high modified Bloom-Richardson scores. In other words, these cancers tend to be fast growing, fast spreading, and aggressive. Basal-type breast cancers are more prevalent in young women, and they often present as a palpable mass. Ninety percent of breast cancer in women who have a *BRCA1* gene mutation is the basal type, compared to fourteen percent in *BRCA2* carriers (see chapter 11).

The triple-negative type of breast cancer has received much attention from researchers. Breast cancer cells are most sensitive to chemotherapeutic agents when the cells are actively reproducing and growing. As previously noted, triple-negative cancer cells are highly active, and because of their high proliferation rate they are quite sensitive to chemotherapy. The treatment of triple-negative cancers is evolving with the discovery of new agents and methods to deliver them. (This is further discussed in chapter 10.)

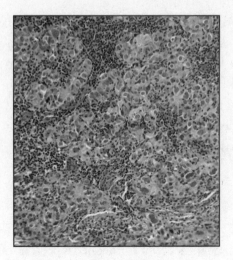

Figure 3.4
Basal-type or triple-negative

HER2-Positive Breast Cancer

✌ Approximately 15 percent of breast cancers overproduce a gene called the *HER2 oncogene* (a gene that causes cancer). This oncogene promotes the growth of cancer cells by sending messages to the cells to grow and to spread. Cancers that are positive for the HER2 oncogene tend to be more aggressive than other types of breast cancer, and they are either hormone-positive or hormone-negative, which will influence decisions about future hormone treatment. These fast- growing cancers have high Ki67 and high-modified Bloom-Richardson scores. Like basal-type breast cancer, this type is more prevalent in younger women and is usually found as a rapidly growing breast mass. Diagnosis of HER2-positive breast cancer depends on identifying the presence of *HER2 receptors* on the cell surface using a special *immunohistochemical* (IHC) test, a process that stains the receptors so that they are easier to see under the microscope (Figures 3.5a and 3.5b).

The IHC staining provides a score of 0, 1, 2, or 3, based on the number of HER2 receptors that are seen on the cell surface. Zero and 1 are

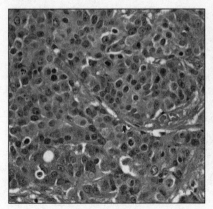
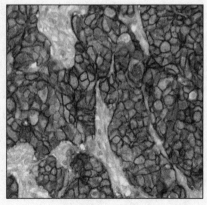

Figure 3.5a
HER2-positive

Figure 3.5b
HER2-positive with IHC staining

considered *negative* for HER2 oncogene, while 3 is positive for overproduction of HER2. A 2 is *indeterminate* and requires an additional test to measure the HER2 oncogene *inside* the cell using a fluorescent stain known as *fluorescence in situ hybridization (FISH)*. A third method that measures gene overactivity, known as *reverse transcription*-polymerase chain reaction (RT-PCR), is now commercially available. It is critical to accurately determine if a breast cancer produces the HER2 receptor because a highly effective therapy has been specifically developed to treat this type of cancer. (The therapy is not effective with other breast cancers.)

The tremendous progress made in the treatment of HER2-positive breast cancer is due to our increased understanding of the *molecular pathways* within the cell and the development of chemical agents that can disrupt the pathways. An antibody to the HER2 receptor (Herceptin), when added to chemotherapy, has greatly increased the cure rate for HER2-positive breast cancer (chapter 7). Further understanding of the *intracellular* (inside the cell) pathways has led to the discovery of additional targeted chemical agents (lapatinib, neratinib) that can block signals within the cells, causing the cells to die. To me, this is one of the most exciting areas of breast cancer treatment—understanding the molecular basis of the malignant process that can lead to the development of targeted treatments capable of reversing the process.

The new classification replaces the previous one, which divided breast cancers into two cell types: *invasive ductal carcinoma* and *infiltrating lobular carcinoma*. Ductal cancer can be any of the four cell types, but lobular falls into the Luminal B category. Ductal cancers originate in the duct just before the duct ends in the *lobule*. Lobules are *globes* of glandular cells that produce milk, and it is believed that lobular cancers originated from these cells. As discussed in chapter 1, the beginnings of cancer can remain within the confines of the ductal system—what is termed *in situ*. *Ductal carcinoma in situ* (DCIS) is discussed at length in chapter 7.

Within the lumen of the lobule an in situ lesion can develop that was previously called *lobular carcinoma in situ* (LCIS). Because LCIS actually represents a premalignant condition, it is now referred to as *lobular neoplasia*. Unlike DCIS, the cells inside the lobules do not form calcification. We are not even sure that lobular neoplasia leads to invasive breast cancer. This is an area of ongoing discussion and controversy among the medical and research communities. What we do know is that lobular neoplasia is often associated with infiltrating lobular cancer, but it is not clear that it is the precursor. Lobular neoplasia that is discovered as an incidental finding *with or without* an associated cancer increases a woman's risk of developing breast cancer in the future. This cancer can be any of the four previously described types but is most often associated with Luminal B. The finding of lobular neoplasia is very important in treatment planning and future risk reduction strategies. Table 3.1 demonstrates the characteristics of the new genomic classification of invasive breast cancer.

Medullary Breast Cancer

This is a triple-negative breast cancer that has a prominent immune reaction that looks very high-grade under the microscope. It tends to

New Classification	Hormone Receptors: Estrogen (ER) and Progesterone (PR)	Modified Bloom-Richardson Score	Ki67
Luminal A	Strong for both	low	low
Luminal B	ER is positive, PR is often weak	intermediate	intermediate
Basal-type	Negative	high	high
HER2-positive	Positive or negative	high	high

Table 3.1

New classification of breast cancer

occur in younger women and is very scary because it has a high prolif-eration rate since the cancer cells are very high-grade. But there is a prominent immune reaction with lymphocytes (immune cells) sur-rounding the cancer. I have treated perhaps twenty young women with medullary breast cancer using chemotherapy, and they all sur-vived. Later in chapter 10 we will discuss triple-negative breast cancer and genomic subtypes. Medullary, triple-negative breast cancer is labeled by its appearance under the microscope, but I suspect it has a unique genetic mutation that activates the immune system. Fortunately, it has a very good prognosis.

Cystosarcoma Phyllodes

✣ This unusual tumor can be noncancerous or malignant. The dis-tinction can be difficult for the pathologist to make. This cancer's pre-sentation is usually that of an enlarging mass in the breast of a young woman. Clinically and on scans and other imaging, the lump usually looks and feels like a benign tumor known as a fibroadenoma, a com-mon occurrence in young women. However, these lesions can grow large and grow rapidly, unlike fibroadenomas, which seldom exceed 2 centimeters. When the healthy cell converts into its malignant form, it resembles a sarcoma; it does not spread to lymph nodes, and it does not involve the duct system. The malignant form rarely spreads into the blood system.

The treatment of choice is surgery, and lymph node sampling is not necessary. Patients with large tumors, which make breast conservation impossible without major deformity, should consider a skin-sparing type of mastectomy with immediate reconstruction. In our experience, the nipple and areola can be spared because cystosarcoma phyllodes tumors do not involve the ducts. The role of chemotherapy and radiation therapy in the malignant form is not clear. These cancers are not of glandular origin and are really sarcomas.

Metaplastic Breast Cancer

This breast cancer is a rare form of triple-negative breast cancer and is discussed in chapter 10. Under the microscope, metaplastic breast cancer is unique in that it has characteristics of non-breast-cancer types. It can have areas of the cancer that look like squamous cancer of the lung or areas that resemble cancer of mesenchymal origin like sarcomas of the muscle or cartilage. Almost always triple-negative, it is aggressive and rapidly divides, requiring adjuvant chemotherapy. At Breastlink centers, we send samples of metaplastic breast cancer to laboratories that perform molecular pathway profiling in order to help us select the most appropriate chemotherapy.

Paget's Disease

Paget's disease of the breast presents as a scaly, itchy nipple. It is a persistent problem, and often women first seek medical help from a dermatologist. Paget's disease is an in situ breast cancer of the nipple ducts that is frequently associated with underlying invasive breast cancer (approximately 50 percent of the time). This possibility should be carefully investigated. The treatment of choice is a wide excision of the nipple-areolar complex.

Inflammatory Breast Cancer

❧ Inflammatory breast cancer (IBC) mimics infection of the breast (mastitis) and does not respond to antibiotics. It is an aggressive cancer that is usually triple-negative and spreads rapidly through the lymphatic system under the skin of the breast, resulting in what appears to be an angry dermatitis (inflammation of the skin). Diagnosis is often made by a skin biopsy. The treatment for IBC is chemotherapy followed by surgery. This cancer, once almost always fatal, now has a much better prognosis when aggressive systemic chemotherapy is given prior to surgery.

Special Types of Luminal A Breast Cancer: Tubular, Papillary (Mucinous or Colloid), and Cribriform

❧ These variants of Luminal A breast cancer have an excellent prognosis and are treated with surgery. The risk of systemic spread is minimal.

4

· · · · · ·

The Pathology Report

You will want to review and understand your pathology report. Historically, physicians often believed that it was better for patients to have limited access to their medical reports. Doctors wanted to interpret the medical jargon prior to presentation to the patient because they were concerned that patients might misunderstand the information contained in the report. This thinking has changed among the medical community today. The philosophy at our breast centers and at many others is that it is important for you to read and understand your pathology report, even if it contains confusing or bad news. We want to help you understand the meaning of this health information so that you can become an integral part of your own health team. Our group has worked closely with breast pathologists to develop and format a report that provides consistent and meaningful information. When we conduct a second opinion, we review a patient's tissue slides and corresponding pathology report, which includes a written description of the tissue received in the laboratory (called a *macroscopic* or *gross* description).

Most women today will have at least two separate pathology reports. The first is usually from the diagnostic needle biopsy of the cancer, and the second is generated from the breast surgery that follows at a later date. If the cancer is not *palpable* (cannot be felt), the needle biopsy will be obtained using image guidance such as ultrasound or MRI. Information collected from imaging coupled with the biopsy results will give the treating team important information about planning further treatment.

Historically, the pathology report was a written description of what the pathologist observed when looking at the cancer tissue under the microscope. Usually this was the surgical biopsy tissue from a mastectomy or partial mastectomy. The pathologist described the nature of the cancer cells or how similar or dissimilar they were from a normal cell (*their degree of differentiation*), the total size of the cancer, whether there appeared to be invasion into the surrounding blood vessels or lymph system, and if there appeared to be any reaction or response to the cancer by the patient's own defense system (*host response*). Usually included along with the surgical specimen were the regional lymph nodes, and the pathologist carefully examined slices of each node to determine if the cancer had spread.

From this information the cancer was staged (stage 1, 2, or 3 *or* TNM staging), and it was decided whether radiation was needed. When chemotherapy became available in the late 1970s, information from the pathologic review was critical to ascertain the need for its use. Because of limited options in the early era of breast cancer treatment, the pathologic description of the breast tissue was primarily evaluated to predict patient outcome (*prognosis*). As more sophisticated and innovative therapies and technologies were developed, the pathologic analysis evolved into a health management tool that was able to drive the decision-making around treatment options that would influence a woman's chance for a cure.

While the early analyses presented information that to this day is the bedrock of the pathology report, new developments added to and enhanced our knowledge of the unique aspects of the cancer cell to help us understand the individual patient's cancer characteristics. One major development was the discovery of specialized receptors on the cancer cell surface that soon became targets for therapy. Techniques were developed using special stains that identified the presence or absence of *hormone receptors* on the cancer cell surface. These first *immunohistochemical stains* (IHC) were designed to identify estrogen and progesterone receptors. The presence or absence of the receptors predicted whether hormonal therapies would be effective in controlling the cancer. Indeed, clinical trials did prove that hormonal agents such as tamoxifen and the aromatase inhibitors could effectively kill this type of cancer cell in women whose cancer tested positive for hormone receptors (see chapter 8).

Much later another type of receptor was found in an especially aggressive breast cancer. Originally called the *epidermal growth factor receptor*, this receptor is now known as the *HER2 receptor*. This development led to the discovery of an important therapeutic drug known as Herceptin that is specifically directed at this receptor. HER2 receptors test results (and most likely others in the future) are now an extremely important part of the information contained within the pathology report, and they are absolutely critical in the modern treatment of breast cancer.

Most recently we have entered a new era of *genomic analysis* of cancer cells. Results from this testing are rapidly being incorporated into treatment planning. Investigators are now able to examine genetic differences among cancers and identify genes that are associated with invasion, spread, aggressiveness, and metastasis. We are in the early days of these types of analyses, but we can already examine tumor tissue to identify women who are likely to relapse and who will therefore benefit from chemotherapy. Equally important, genetic analysis of this type identifies women who will *not* benefit from chemotherapy, thus preventing unnecessary treatment with the associated side effects. Because we have only just entered the realm of genomic analysis, the highly specialized testing is performed in a limited number of laboratories.

Today's pathology report still contains the physical description of the cancer and the measurement of its size. Based on new and innovative research developments, the pathology report also states whether cell surface receptors are present or absent and often provides the results of genomic analysis. In the future we can expect that the pathology report will include all of this and more. We cannot emphasize enough that accurate and thorough pathology reporting is critical to predicting outcome and prognosis. Planning appropriate treatment based on the pathology report will result in increased patient survival.

Now that we have discussed the important role that the pathology report plays in your diagnosis and treatment, I want to help you read and understand your own pathology report.

Pathology Report: Needle Biopsy

✂ Ninety percent of newly diagnosed women will receive a breast cancer diagnosis based on a needle biopsy resulting from detection of a palpable breast lump or from an abnormality identified by mammogram. The biopsy is a small cylinder of tissue the diameter of a pencil lead and about 5 millimeters long. Even though it is very small, the pathologist is able to obtain a tremendous amount of information about the cancer from the needle biopsy, and this information is formally presented on the pathology report (see Figure 4.1). The report may differ somewhat from laboratory to laboratory; however, the information presented is fairly standard across institutions and will most likely contain the following sections:

Patient identifying information
Final diagnosis
Microscopic description
Molecular studies
Clinical and gross description
Pathologist signature and date of review
Signature of confirming pathologist review

Hill Crest Hospital   (999)999-9999   George C. Scott, M.D., Lab Director
Patient name: Maxine Libby
MR# AB12345678   DOB: 01/01/1956
Specimen #: P-7777-23   Date collected: 06/09/2016   Received in lab: 06/09/2016
Specimen type: BREAST BIOPSY, NEEDLE

Final Diagnosis
(Microscopic)

Right Breast, Core Biopsy: —Infiltrating Ductal Carcinoma, High-Grade

Summary for invasive breast carcinoma in core biopsy

Anatomic location: Right Breast (12:00)

Needle Biopsy Guidance: Core Biopsy (NOS)

Result for Surgery: Irregular Mass

Imaging Size of lesion: 1.8 cm
                                      (Pathologic tumor size deferred to excisional specimens)

Histologic Type: Infiltrating ductal carcinoma

Tumor Grade: SBR 8/9 (high)
                              -Tubules: 3/3
                              -Nuclear grade: 3/3
                              -Mitosis: 2/3

Prognostic Markers: Performed

Ductal Carcinoma in Situ: Not present

Microcalcifications: Not identified

Lymphatic invasion: Absent

Molecular Studies
Breast Cancer Prognostic Markers

Specimen: Formalin fixed, paraffin block 0

Procedure: Immunohistochemistry, LSAB detection method

Assay: Estrogen Receptors
        Results: Negative   Favorable result: Positive 1–3+

Assay: Progesterone Receptors
        Results: Negative   Favorable result: Positive 1–3+

Assay: HER2/neu
        Results: Negative, 1+ Favorable result: Negative 0–1+

Clinical

Pre-op diagnosis: Right breast, 12 o'clock, irregular mass 1.8 cm

Post-op diagnosis: Suspect malignant

Gross Description:

Labeled right breast is a 1.2 x 0.5 x 0.2 cm aggregate of yellow-tan fibrofatty tissue.
Formalin fixation time, 9 hours.

Signed: Dr. Steven R. Johnson   **Date:** 06/10/16

Findings reviewed and confirmed by: Dr. Frank Wong   **Date:** 06/11/16

Figure 4.1

Sample pathology report from needle biopsy

The pathologist will observe the tissue under the microscope and determine if the cancer is confined to the ducts (DCIS) or if it has invaded through the basement membrane of the ducts into the surrounding tissue to become an invasive (or infiltrating) breast cancer. If the pathologist interprets the biopsy as entirely ductal carcinoma in situ (DCIS), the report will be moderately different than if there is invasion present. DCIS and its pathologic characteristics and treatments are thoroughly discussed in chapter 7. The focus of this chapter will be the pathology report for an invasive breast cancer. If the breast cancer has been found to be invasive, the pathologist will determine the grade of the cancer. *Grade* is defined as the degree of malignancy— how far the cells have changed from the original normal cell (or the cell of origin). The pathologist uses a scaling system called the *modified Bloom-Richardson scale* (MBR) to determine the grade. Three separate characteristics of the cancer cells will be examined: (1) the amount of tubule formation, (2) the nuclear size, and (3) the number of cells in active cell division (*mitosis*). The MBR system assigns a score of 1 to 3 for *each* characteristic, with 1 being least, or smallest, and 3 being most, or largest. A minimum score of 3 and a maximum score of 9 can be achieved with this system. In Table 4.1 this cancer is given a 2 for tubule formation, a 2 for nuclear size, and a 1 for mitotic rate. This results in a total score of 5 out of a possible 9, written as 5/9. This score is consistent with a Luminal A breast cancer as depicted in Figure 3.2 in chapter 3.

Tumor cell characteristics	1	2	3
Tubule formation		X	
Nuclear size		X	
Mitotic rate	X		

Table 4.1
Determining total MBR score

Scores of 3, 4, or 5 are considered low-grade, 6 or 7 are intermediate-grade, and 8 or 9 are high-grade cancers (Table 4.2). As described in the previous example, an MBR score of 5 is consistent with a low-grade breast cancer. The next task for the pathologist is to describe the cancer cells and their patterns as seen under the microscope. Pathologists traditionally have segregated breast cancers into ductal versus lobular patterns. This distinction is still important because lobular cancers have unique characteristics. They tend to be larger than they appear on the breast images, they tend to have satellite foci (which may appear as individual specks), and they are often associated with an increased incidence of a second cancer in the future. Lobular cancers fall into the Luminal B group in the new classification (chapter 3). Under the microscope they do not form tubules, and they appear to branch, or "flow," into the fat and supporting tissue in the surrounding breast. Lobular cancers are hormone-positive and HER2-negative almost without exception. A special stain called *e-cahedrin*, when applied to the biopsy tissue, can help the pathologist distinguish between ductal and lobular carcinomas.

The pathologist will sometimes describe special patterns of growth or arrangement of the cancer cells such as *papillary* or *cribriform* or *tubular*, which are, I believe, somewhat outdated terms having little relevance today. These three tend to be subsets of low-grade ductal cancers (chapter 3).

Grade	MBR Score
Low (1)	3, 4, 5
Intermediate (2)	6, 7
High (3)	8, 9

Table 4.2

Determining tumor grade using the MBR score

More important is the description of whether the cancer cells have invaded the lymph or vascular structures, information that is associated with increased spread to the lymph nodes and that has important treatment implications.

Next the pathologist can perform tests in which different stains are put on thin slices of the needle biopsy, and which give the treating team useful information for making treatment decisions. This technique, called *immunohistochemical staining* (IHC), is able to detect the presence of specific proteins within the cell and on the cell surface.

The four most common IHC tests identify:

1. estrogen receptors
2. progesterone receptors
3. HER2
4. Ki67

The hormone receptors and HER2 receptor tests aid in the selection of targeted treatment options and help to determine the cancer type. The Ki67 test identifies cancer cells that are preparing to divide. The percentage of cells that are positive for Ki67 determines how rapidly the cancer is growing (proliferation rate). In other words, a high Ki67 score usually indicates a fast-growing cancer.

Results from the pathologist review are so critically important to the decision-making and treatment planning that most laboratories require an independent second review to confirm the diagnosis of cancer. The important information obtained from the biopsy, combined with that from imaging and the clinical exam, provides the framework for treatment planning. Even more information about the cancer can be obtained by sending a portion of the biopsy to specialized laboratories for further gene analysis. This testing identifies whether genes within the cell involved in cell proliferation, invasion, and metabolic spread are active.

Presently, there are a few companies that commercially perform this type of testing. At Breastlink we use two commercial companies to perform this gene testing in breast cancer. Agendia performs a seventy-gene analysis, or assay, that is called MammaPrint. The second company, Genomic Health, performs a twenty-one-gene assay called Oncotype DX. Both of these tests are used in the case of Luminal cancers to determine increased risk of systemic spread and the need for chemotherapy. I suspect that more of these gene tests will become available in the near future as our knowledge of the malignant process expands. Not only will these tests predict the risk of systemic spread, but they will identify which targeted drugs should be used.

Pathology Report: Surgical

✇ The second pathology report occurs following the surgical removal of the cancer. This surgery may be a *wide local excision* (WLE), also known as a *lumpectomy*, or it may be a mastectomy. Often the surgery involves removal of one or more lymph nodes (see chapter 6). A course of preoperative (neoadjuvant) chemotherapy may occur before either of these surgeries, which can greatly alter the extent and appearance of the cancer. It is not uncommon for there to be no cancer remaining at the time of surgery, which is called a *pathologic complete response* (pCR).

A pathologic complete response is much more common in the triple-negative and HER2 types of breast cancer. The surgical pathology report describes the size of the invasive cancer and the associated in situ cancer, if any. It notes the presence or absence of lymph node involvement and provides details on the cancer cells' appearance under the microscope, along with the MBR grade. If IHC stains were not performed on the needle biopsy, they can be performed now for estrogen and progesterone receptors, HER2 receptors, and Ki67. The surgical pathology report may include information from the prior needle biopsy. (Figure 4.2 is a sample surgical pathology report.)

The goal of surgery is to remove the cancer completely plus a rim of normal tissue around it. When the surgeon removes the cancer s/he

Hill Crest Hospital (999)999-9999 George C. Scott, M.D., Lab Director Page 1 of 2
Patient name: Maxine Libby
MR# AB12345678 DOB: 01/01/1956

Specimen #: P-7777-23 Date collected: 06/09/2016 Received in lab: 06/09/2016
Specimen type: Partial mastectomy

Final Diagnosis
(Microscopic)

Right Breast, Partial mastectomy: Infiltrating Ductal Carcinoma, High Grade
Summary for invasive breast carcinoma in partial mastectomy
Anatomic location: Right Breast (12:00)
Size of specimen: 6 x 5 x 5 cm
Size of tumor: 1.8 cm
Histologic Type: Infiltrating ductal carcinoma, high-grade
Tumor Grade: MBR 8/9 (high)
-Tubules: 3/3
-Nuclear grade: 3/3
-Mitosis: 2/3
Tumor necrosis: Not present
Margins of resection: Free of tumor
Prognostic Markers: Performed
Stage: $T_{1c}N_{1a}$
Nipple involvement: NA
Ductal Carcinoma in Situ: Not present
Microcalcifications: None
Lymph nodes: 1/11 nodes positive for cancer

Molecular Studies
Breast Cancer Prognostic Markers
Specimen: Formalin fixed, paraffin block 0
Procedure: Immunohistochemistry, LSAB detection method
Assay: Estrogen Receptors
Results: Negative Favorable result: Positive 1–3+
Assay: Progesterone Receptors
Results: Negative Favorable result: Positive 1–3+
Assay: HER2/neu
Results: Negative, 1+ Favorable result: Negative 0–1+

Clinical
Pre-op diagnosis: Right breast cancer
Specimen(s)

A. Right breast tissue
B. Right axillary contents

Gross Description:

A. Is received fresh, labeled "right breast mass" fatty tissue measuring 6 x 5 x 5 cm.

Signed: Dr. Steven R. Johnson **Date:** 06/10/16
Findings reviewed and confirmed by: Dr. Frank Wong **Date:** 06/11/16

Figure 4.2

Sample surgical pathology report

Tumor size	
T_0	In situ (with no invasion)
$T_{1a}, T_{1b},$ or T_{1c}	1a: 0–5 mm, 1b: 5–10 mm, 1c: 10–20 mm
T_2	20–50 mm
T_3	>50 mm
T_4	Invasion into the skin or underlying muscle
Lymph node involvement	
N_0	No node involvement
N_{1a}	1–3 nodes involved
N_{1b}	4–10 nodes involved
N_{1c}	>10 nodes involved
Distant spread	
M_x	Unknown if cancer spread to distant site
M_0	No spread to distant site
M_+	Cancer spread to a distant site

Table 4.3

TNM staging

orients it for the pathologist using small clips. The pathologist examines the removed specimen under the microscope and determines if there is clearance of normal tissue completely surrounding the cancer (clear margins) and to what extent (measurement in mm). This information is presented on the pathology report under *Margins of resection*. Included in the surgical pathology report is the stage of the breast cancer. The staging system involves the extent of the primary cancer and the spread to the lymph nodes. This system is called the *TNM system*, where T is tumor size, N is number of lymph nodes, and M is metastatic disease (spread to another part of the body). (Figure 4.3 describes the TNM strategy.) Historically, the TNM staging system was correlated to prognosis and survival, but today I believe it has less relevance.

This system does not take into consideration the biology or aggressiveness of the cancer, which is more important in prognosis than the extent of disease. Women who receive preoperative chemotherapy will never have an accurate pathologic staging of their cancer because treatment will alter what the pathologist will ultimately see under the microscope.

5
. . . . . .
✌

Local Control

The cure of breast cancer depends on two types of control: *local control* and *systemic control*. We will discuss systemic control in chapter 6. Local control is defined as the complete removal of the primary cancer in the breast and any secondary spread to the adjacent lymph nodes in the axilla (armpit). The objective of local control is to remove the cancer in its entirety. Fifty years ago the only approach was to remove the entire breast—a mastectomy. As screening mammography discovered smaller cancers, clinical trials conducted in the 1970s and 1980s demonstrated that local control could be achieved with less surgery—surgery that is called a *lumpectomy, partial mastectomy,* or *wide local excision* (WLE). We will use the later term throughout the rest of the manual.

Two major research trials, one in Italy and the other in the United States, proved that WLE in conjunction with radiation for smaller cancers gave equal local control when compared to mastectomy. Women treated with WLE without radiation had approximately a 30 percent local recurrence rate. These patients with recurrences required a mastectomy; however, there was no decrease in the cure rate. (We discuss radiation therapy added to WLE later in this chapter.) At the time of mastectomy or WLE, the regional lymph nodes in the axilla were removed. (Figure 1.5 in chapter 1 demonstrates the breast lymph node drainage.) It was thought that local control required removal of a majority of lymph nodes located in the axilla of the involved breast. This standard lymph node procedure removed the first two levels of nodes— approximately ten to twenty in number. Many women were found to have no cancerous involvement in the removed nodes, and approximately 10 percent of the women developed permanent swelling of their arm (*lymphedema*). It was discovered that removal of the nodes at the time of initial surgery did not increase the cure rate, but the presence of cancer cells in one or more nodes predicted an increase in systemic spread and became an important factor in selecting women who would benefit from adding systemic therapy to the surgery.

The next important advance was the discovery that breast cancer usually spreads to a single node, called the *sentinel lymph node*, before continuing into adjacent nodes in the region. It was found that the sentinel node could be identified by injecting a special dye and/or a radioactive tracer into or around the cancer prior to surgery. The surgeon is then able to isolate the location of the sentinel node using a radioactivity-sensing probe and with a small incision; the sentinel node is identified by its blue color. This procedure is performed when there are no obvious abnormal lymph nodes discovered in physical exam or ultrasound imaging. The node is then removed at the time of the WLE or mastectomy for analysis, and if no cancer cells are present, no further lymph node removal is necessary. The incidence of lymphedema has dramatically decreased because of this procedure.

More recent clinical trials have demonstrated that even with a positive sentinel lymph node, extensive removal of additional nodes is not necessary. Since one of the criteria for systemic therapy is the spread to the sentinel lymph node, a positive node will initiate the need for systemic therapy. Recent studies indicate that systemic therapy treats the remaining lymph nodes as well as the rest of the body and the incidence of local recurrence in the axilla is the same as that following surgical removal of the remaining lymph nodes.

The past fifty years of clinical research studies in the local control of breast cancer form the basis for our present treatment decisions and are summarized below:

- WLE with radiation is equal to mastectomy for local control in women with T1 and T2 breast cancers (cancers less than 5 cm).
- Radiation reduces the risk of local recurrence but does not increase the cure rate.
- In women with no clinical evidence of lymph node involvement, removal of an uninvolved sentinel lymph node predicts there is no spread of cancer to the remaining axillary lymph nodes.
- Women with larger cancers (greater than 5 cm) are not good candidates for WLE and require mastectomy. Recent studies demonstrate that systemic therapy administrated prior to surgery will often reduce the size of the cancer and allow for breast conservation.
- Women with cancers greater than 5 centimeters and with multiple lymph nodes involved have an increased local recurrence rate even with mastectomy and therefore benefit from radiation.

Because of this progress, the number of women receiving mastectomy and extensive lymph node removal has been greatly reduced. The number of women cured of breast cancer in the past thirty years has greatly increased, but this has little to do with the extent of surgery. Local control is necessary and very important, but with good preoperative planning, less surgery is needed. The increase in cure rate is largely due to earlier diagnosis (a result of earlier detection) and more effective systemic therapy (discussed in the next chapter).

In performing a WLE, the breast surgeon should remove the cancer in its entirety with a rim of normal breast tissue surrounding the cancer—what is called an "uninvolved margin." The amount of deformity and volume loss depends on the location of the cancer in the breast and the size of the cancer plus the uninvolved margins. If the cancer is in close proximity to the skin, skin may need to be resected. The goal is to remove the cancer completely with clear margins leaving a breast that is cosmetically acceptable. In recent years, dedicated breast cancer surgeons have developed techniques that better accomplish this goal. These techniques, called *oncoplastic surgery*, involve moving remaining breast tissue around to repair defects, reducing the volume of the opposite breast to give symmetry, or having assistance from a plastic (reconstructive) surgeon to add volume with silicone implants or fat transfer.

I should mention that despite this progress, over the last many years there has been an increase in the mastectomy rate—particularly among women opting for *bilateral mastectomy* (removal of both breasts). Some of this increase is a result of our ability to identify women with hereditary germ line mutations that put them at increased risk of a second or third breast cancer. Some women choose mastectomy to avoid radiation despite the evidence supporting the benefits of radiation. The progress in reconstruction surgery with nipple and skin sparing has made mastectomy a more acceptable option to women considering it (to be discussed later in this chapter).

Systemic therapy, which we will discuss in the next chapter, has a role in local control. If a woman receives systemic therapy (either chemotherapy or hormonal therapy) prior to surgery, it is called *preoperative*, or *neoadjuvant*, systemic therapy. The first trials of preoperative chemotherapy focused on women with locally advanced cancers that couldn't be completely removed using surgery or women with a rare form of breast cancer involving the skin lymphatics, called *inflammatory breast cancer*, and surgery likewise couldn't entirely remove the cancer. It was discovered that by giving systemic chemotherapy prior to surgery, the cancer would often dramatically shrink and allow for successful surgical removal. The use of preoperative (neoadjuvant) chemotherapy and hormonal therapy is now commonly used in stage 2 and stage 3 breast cancer to reduce the size of the cancer and the extent of lymph node involvement. This allows for less deforming surgery: fewer mastectomies and less extensive lymph node removals are needed. There are other advantages of preoperative systemic therapy, to be discussed in the next chapter.

Radiation Therapy in Local Control

❦ As we discussed in the previous section, radiation is a local treatment added to surgical removal of the breast cancer and is used to prevent local recurrence. It is administered by physician specialists known as radiation oncologists. Radiation therapy is usually given with a large machine called a linear accelerator that generates a high-energy X-ray beam used to treat a specific, well-defined area of the body, or it can be administered using radioactive seeds temporarily placed in the cancer site. Radiation affects the tissue cells beneath the directed beam of X-rays. Cells that are dividing are more affected by radiation than resting cells. Although both cancer and normal cells are damaged by radiation, cancer cells are most affected because they are actively dividing. In addition, normal cells have a greater ability than cancer cells to repair themselves following radiation exposure. Radiation puts cancer cells into a death cycle, called apoptosis, the next time the cancer cell divides.

Many of our patients do not clearly understand the role that radiation therapy plays in the overall treatment plan. For instance, some wonder why radiation is necessary if a breast cancer has been removed by a wide local excision (WLE) with clear margins. As discussed previously, despite local removal with clear margins, about 30 percent of women will relapse locally without radiation therapy, whereas 5 percent or less who receive radiation will relapse. Pathologists can have trouble determining if there is a clear margin of normal tissue surrounding the cancer because it is often difficult to identify minuscule amounts of cancer cells. There may also be "skip" areas between the main tumor and very small, hard-to-detect satellite cancer nodules in the immediate vicinity. Therefore, in spite of clear margins, extremely small tumor cells may be resting on the outside of the surgical margins. In addition, cells may have traveled through the breast duct system and come to rest outside of the surgical site. Radiation is important because it has a good chance of destroying those undetected cancer cells.

Radiation to the chest surface is sometimes also recommended following mastectomy if the cancer is large or has extended to or through the surgical margins or if multiple lymph nodes are involved with cancer. The addition of radiation in these situations reduces the incidence of local recurrence considerably.

Is radiation always necessary? If we could pick the 70 to 80 percent of women who would not have a local recurrence, we could avoid radiation in the majority of cases. Unfortunately, this is not so easy to do. If the cancer is small, with a large clear margin of uninvolved tissue and if there is no local involvement in the lymph nodes or extensive DCIS, one might consider observation alone and no radiation.

Studies also indicate that a woman's age may be an important contributing factor for risk of local recurrence if radiation therapy is not administered. Dr. Umberto Veronesi, who was a world-renowned Italian breast surgeon, reported results from a study in which women with small T1 breast cancers (less than 20 mm) received wide local excision with clear surgical margins. Each woman was then randomly assigned to either postoperative radiation or no radiation. Women over the age of sixty had less than a 5 percent recurrence rate without radiation! Younger women had a higher local recurrence rate without radiation for reasons that are not clear. These findings have led to further studies in the United States confirming that older women (over the age of seventy) with early breast cancer can be spared radiation, particularly if they are receiving hormonal therapy.

The typical course of radiation is daily treatment for twenty-five to thirty sessions. There is good reason to give such extended, prolonged treatment. A long string of short, individual treatments causes less damage to normal tissues, allowing them to repair completely while increasing the progressive lethal damage to cancer cells. Recent studies suggest that it is safe and feasible to reduce the number of treatments to three weeks (fifteen total treatments). This course of radiation, called hypofractionated or accelerated whole breast radiation, reduces the number of treatments but increases the dose of each treatment. A large study in Canada of 2,500 women who received the reduced number of treatments showed no difference in local recurrence or survival rate compared to the traditional thirty treatments with only minor differences in skin reaction and fatigue.

Receiving radiation treatments involves several steps. First, you will have a consultation with the radiation oncologist, who will explain the risks and benefits of the treatment in detail. If radiation is to be part of treatment, the next step is a treatment planning session, called a *simulation* appointment, which can take one to two hours. Most radiation facilities use three-dimensional images from a special CT scanner called a CT simulator to plan treatments. During simulation, the radiation staff will position your body on the CT scanner in the appropriate treatment position—typically lying on your back with one or both arms resting over your head. They will use special devices such as an incline board or customized body pillow to maximize the comfort and reproducibility of your body position.

To ensure accurate positioning prior to each radiation treatment, photographs are taken and small tattoos (the size of a beauty mark) and felt-pen marks are placed on your skin. Stickers and tape may also be used to outline scars and protect ink marks. A CT scan of your body in the treatment position is then sent to the radiation-planning computers. Over the next week, the radiation oncologist will work with a staff physicist to create a radiation treatment plan for you. The images from your simulation are used to target the radiation beam and calculate parameters for the linear accelerator to deliver the correct dose of radiation to your breast. When the treatment plan has been reviewed, approved, and has passed quality assurance checks, your radiation treatments will begin. The radiation machine, called a linear accelerator, is large and imposing (Figure 5.1), and for the minute or two that you are being treated, you may feel alone. My patients say the first treatment is the "scary one" and then there is nothing to it.

The daily treatment appointment is typically fifteen to thirty minutes. Most of that time is spent setting up and verifying the treatment position. The radiation beam is typically on for only one to two minutes, and it comes from two to three different directions. As with a chest X-

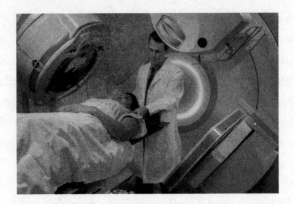

Figure 5.1
Linear accelerator

ray, there is no pain or heat when the radiation beam is passing through the breast. And you will not become radioactive or expose people to radiation during the treatments. The radiation treatments are given by highly trained technicians. Most women will see their radiation oncologist once a week for monitoring, but they should remember that their physician is always available for any special problems that may arise from the daily treatment. Don't hesitate to ask to see the doctor with any questions or concerns you may have.

If the margins around the cancer are surgically clear and the purpose of the radiation is to eradicate any microscopic cells that may have been left behind, fifteen to thirty treatments to the entire breast or chest surface are usually adequate to achieve this goal. However, in younger women, or if the team has some question about margin involvement, an extra amount of radiation, called a boost, is given to the tumor area.

There are several methods of giving boosts. The most common involves the linear accelerator and consists of five to ten additional radiation treatments to the local surgical area using an electron beam. Unlike X-rays used to treat the entire breast, electrons penetrate less deeply into the breast tissue and can be used to target the superficial surgical scar and surgical site just beneath it. Sometimes X-rays are necessary for the boost if your surgical site is deep within a larger-size breast.

There are side effects from radiation to the breast. It is usual to have some skin and breast tissue changes, such as redness and inflammation, which usually diminish over time. Ninety percent of women have an excellent cosmetic result after healing occurs. Ten percent have some added fibrous tissue, shrinkage of the breast, reduced skin elasticity, and breast sensitivity. There are treatments available that can be used to help facilitate healing and reduce the long-term effects of radiation.

Skin side effects must be taken into account when considering reconstruction after mastectomy. Radiation can cause problems with hardening of tissue around breast reconstruction implants or increased firmness in tissue transferred to the chest surface from a TRAM flap, discussed later in this chapter. You should discuss the possible need for radiation therapy with both the oncologist and the plastic surgeon. A consultation with a radiation oncologist prior to mastectomy may be helpful for understanding the potential effects of radiation on a reconstructed breast. In some cases it is better to delay the breast reconstruction until after chemotherapy and radiation therapy so that all choices, with their associated risks and benefits, can be reviewed with you. Some women will have reconstruction at the time of mastectomy, using temporary saline implants that are replaced with permanent implants in a second surgery. If radiation is needed after mastectomy, the second surgery will take place about six months after radiation is completed in order to minimize healing problems due to radiation.

As for other side effects, radiation does pose several. However, with modern techniques the radiation beam is targeted more accurately and thereby avoids excessive radiation to the lungs and heart. The ribs beneath your treated breast may be tender for a year or longer. You may experience temporary fatigue and a mild reduction in white and red blood cell counts. You will not experience nausea or scalp hair loss.

When a woman needs both chemotherapy and radiation, chemotherapy is usually given first. This is because several of the chemotherapy agents raise the toxicity of the radiation and can cause increased skin changes if given along with radiation. Also, if the treatments were to be given at the same time, the bone marrow would suffer a greater impact, resulting in lower white blood cell counts, which can leave a patient more vulnerable to infection.

Many women express concern regarding radiation treatment and its ability to cause other cancers later in life. In order to understand the risk of this possibility, you should know the different sources and types of radiation that humans are exposed to. Some are environmental, such as solar radiation, and are considered "natural," while others are man-made, such as those resulting from X-rays and imaging. It is true that in large doses radiation is carcinogenic and can cause genetic muta-tion. This is often the result of partial injury to a cell that recovers and goes on to divide and pass on defects to offspring cells.

For the most part, these defects do not result from therapeutic ra-diation, thanks to the p53 gene and other DNA-repair genes. The p53 gene is in all cells in the body and appears to protect the cell from most of these mutations. Fortunately, if a cell is injured, the p53 gene pre-vents further cell division until repairs are made. It is amazing that the body has such self-healing potential.

A number of studies have been conducted to determine if there is an increased risk of a second cancer in patients treated with therapeu-tic radiation. Retrospective studies have looked at women receiving pri-mary radiation for the treatment of breast cancer and the incidence of a second breast cancer and other types of malignancy. The bottom line is that there is a very slight increased risk of a second cancer as the result of radiation treatment. Women who have had radiation therapy have approximately a 1 percent chance of getting a second breast can-cer from the treatment itself, compared with women who have not re-ceived radiation in the treatment of their breast cancer. Age seems to be a factor, and the highest risk occurs in women exposed to radiation at a young age. The risk for women over age forty appears to be negli-gible, but not zero.

The use of more limited radiation has been evaluated in clinical trials and is becoming more available and widely adopted. Because breast cancer tends to exist in a specific segment, or quadrant, and local recurrences are usually a centimeter or two from the site of the original cancer, it may be appropriate to limit the extent of radiation; by using radiation seeds or a radiation-filled balloon, the period of radiation exposure may be limited to only five days. This type of radiation, called accelerated partial breast radiation, appears to be appropriate for tumors that are unifocal (isolated to a single area in the breast), small (less than 3 cm), and far enough away from the skin to minimize skin injury. Patients with extensive in situ or lymphatic involvement are not good candidates for this accelerated partial breast radiation because of a higher risk of residual cancer away from the primary cancer. It is appropriate for you to discuss this option with your surgeon and radiation oncologist.

For women who choose to have WLE without radiation, there is an increased risk of local recurrence, as stated above. A majority of these recurrences occur within one to two centimeters of the original tumor resection. This is why localized radiation reduces the incidence of local recurrence. Based on this knowledge, a number of clinical trials around the world have been conducted using a single treatment of radiation administered during the primary surgery. This technique, known as intraoperative radiation (IORT), was pioneered in Italy by Dr. Veronesi. It appears to be effective in preventing local recurrence in women with node-negative cancers that are unifocal and less than 3 centimeters in size. Figure 5.2 shows a patient in the operating room receiving IORT. The advantage of intraoperative radiation is that it is a single treatment and occurs at the same time as the surgery to remove the cancer. If you are a potential candidate for intraoperative radiation based on the above criteria, you may want to inquire about entering into a clinical study using the technique. I believe that in the future intraoperative radiation given at the time of WLE will be the radiation treatment of choice for appropriate patients.

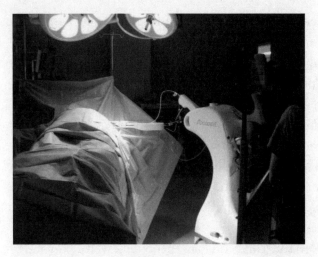

Figure 5.2

Patient receiving intraoperative single-dose radiation

Breast Reconstruction Surgery

✄ Now we are going to discuss reconstruction, a major aspect of optimal local control. It is important that the breast surgeon achieves clear margins, whether a WLE or mastectomy is being performed. The breast surgeon can be more aggressive in achieving clear margins knowing that the defects created can be greatly improved using new reconstructive techniques (known as *oncoplastic surgery*). We are fortunate to have superb plastic surgeons at Breastlink that will partner with our breast surgeons to create the best cosmetic results.

For women diagnosed with either DCIS or invasive breast cancer and who require or desire mastectomy, there has been tremendous progress in the area of breast reconstruction over the last few years. Today the breast cancer surgeon and the plastic reconstruction surgeon work together to form a presurgery plan that results in a far superior outcome compared to earlier attempts at breast reconstruction. The old method involved the plastic surgeon seeing the woman after her mastectomy and attempting to create a reconstruction on a chest wall left with a large scar and limited skin.

In my opinion the present superior and often spectacular results are due to four major developments:

1. Preoperative planning with the breast cancer surgeons and plastic surgeon working together.
2. The emergence of plastic surgeons who specialize in breast reconstruction and who are passionate about what they do.
3. New materials and devices that aid in the reconstruction process.
4. New surgical techniques that often involve skin and even nipple preservation.

The cosmetic result achieved after immediate reconstruction with a skin- and nipple-sparing procedure can be better than that following wide local excision plus radiation. This option eliminates the need for annual surveillance for local recurrence and the five to six weeks required for radiation therapy. At our centers there is an increasing trend in women choosing mastectomy with reconstruction over breast conservation with radiation. If you and your team are considering mastectomy, it is critical that you consult with the plastic surgeon prior to your cancer surgery. These surgical techniques are relatively new and require a high level of coordination and technical skill from the breast surgeon and the plastic surgeon. Don't be afraid to ask the surgical team about the extent of their experience in this type of reconstruction. The best results are achieved when the surgeon has a passion and commitment for the best outcome possible. You may want to ask if it is possible to talk on the phone or in person with women who have had the procedure performed by your surgeon.

There are two basic methods of breast reconstruction. The first involves the use of an *expander,* which is placed beneath the chest muscle (*pectoralis muscle*) at the time of the mastectomy or as a second procedure, depending on patient preference. The chest muscle and skin are then expanded, creating a space that serves as the location for the permanent saline or silicone implant that will be inserted during a second procedure (Figure 5.3). This is the most commonly performed procedure for breast reconstruction in the United States in part because it allows women the most rapid return to their normal activity. Plastic surgeons using newer technology to determine adequate blood flow to the skin flaps and nipple sometimes place the permanent implants at the time of the mastectomy in appropriate candidates.

The second method of breast reconstruction, called a *flap reconstruction*, involves bringing skin and fat to the breast from another area of the body. The usual sites of donor tissue are the patient's tummy (abdomen) or the back. This surgery is more complex and results in an additional scar and site of healing. The advantage of this reconstruction procedure is that it uses a woman's own tissue, eliminating the need for a foreign silicone implant.

There are two techniques for flap reconstruction. The first involves

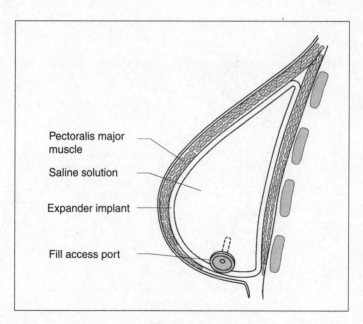

Figure 5.3

Breast reconstruction expander

transferring tissue without disrupting the blood supply (Figure 5.4). This is called a *pedicle transfer* and involves freeing tissue in the abdomen and transferring it to the reconstruction site through a tunnel created by the surgeon beneath the skin. The purpose for moving the abdominal tissue through the tunnel is so that it will retain its intact blood supply with little risk of tissue *necrosis*. The procedure from the abdomen is called a *TRAM* (*Transverse Rectus Abdominis Myocutaneous*). A similar procedure can be done from the back using the *latissimus* muscle. The reason that muscle must be transferred with the overlying fat is that they share a blood supply. The second technique involves removing fat and tissue from the body along with their blood vessels, transferring these to the new site, and reconnecting the blood vessels to existing blood vessels at the new site.

Termed a *free tissue transfer* (*free TRAM* or *DIEP* flap), this procedure

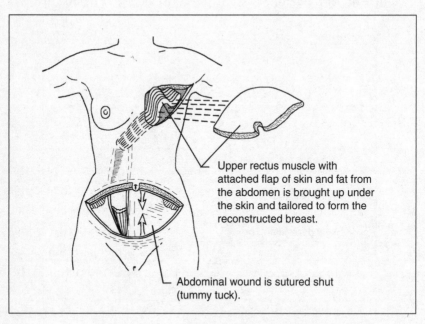

Upper rectus muscle with attached flap of skin and fat from the abdomen is brought up under the skin and tailored to form the reconstructed breast.

Abdominal wound is sutured shut (tummy tuck).

Figure 5.4

Breast reconstruction—tissue transfer

is usually done using the patient's abdominal tissue, and in many cases little muscle needs to be transferred. Special microvascular techniques are required, and the plastic surgeon should specialize in the procedure. This procedure is complex and includes risk of tissue necrosis. It also requires a number of days in the hospital. The advantage over the TRAM procedure is that there is less deformity from the procedure and much less muscle is removed from the abdomen. There are advantages and disadvantages with both reconstruction methods, and it is important to discuss these with your physician.

Decisions about the type of reconstruction are based upon the cancer operation itself (the extent of skin removed and the location of scars) and the amount of fat available to be transferred. A majority of women at our centers undergo expander-type reconstruction. On the whole it is a less complex procedure, and when the surgeons can preserve skin and even the nipple, the result is excellent. In the past, there has been controversy about the use of silicone at the reconstruction site. Based on extensive studies, the FDA has concluded that the current generation of silicone implants is safe and durable. A potential cosmetic problem of expander reconstruction is the coverage of tissue and skin over the silicone implant. If the coverage is too thin, there can be problems with healing (*flap necrosis*) or the results can be less than natural, with visible ripples. The key is for the cancer surgeon to make the skin flaps thick enough with underlying subcutaneous fat to cover the implant without leaving breast glandular tissue. Leaving glandular breast tissue behind increases the risk of a future cancer or a recurrence, while a layer of subcutaneous fat that is too thin can result in a less than acceptable outcome. This is where the experience and skill of the breast surgeon are critical. Plastic surgeons today often combine additional procedures during reconstruction to optimize the results of implant reconstruction.

Many surgeons utilize sheets of protein called *acellular dermal matrix* to add more protective coverage over implants while obtaining a more cosmetically appealing result. Some surgeons will even combine the back-flap procedure (*latissimus*) with expander reconstruction to allow better coverage and more volume. The reconstruction plan is tailored to the individual patient's goals and needs.

The new era of breast reconstruction has given women who require or desire one or more mastectomies excellent cosmetic results. Some women who are prime candidates for WLE with radiation are choosing mastectomy instead to reduce the risk of future breast cancers and to alleviate continued surveillance and potential biopsies. For those women who decide to have breast preservation with WLE, surgeons are now using reconstructive techniques at the time of the surgery, with improved cosmetic results. These techniques, termed *oncoplastic surgery*, involve special approaches to remove the cancer and rearrange the remaining breast tissue to give superior cosmetic outcomes. This often involves some surgery to the unaffected breast as well to provide balance and symmetry.

In summary, we have come a very long way since the radical mastectomy. Our goal now, as it was then, is to achieve local control and remove all cancer from the breast. With spectacular new surgical techniques, women can go on with their lives after breast cancer surgery feeling whole and self-confident and without compromising their chance to be cured. This requires that you understand and discuss these aspects of your care with the surgical members of your treatment team.

6

. . . . . .

Systemic Control

In contrast to *local control* (within your breast), *systemic control* refers to therapies that treat your whole body. Systemic breast cancer treatment involves drugs, antibodies, proteins, and hormones that target breast cancer cells found anywhere in the body. These therapies are usually taken orally, intravenously, or by intramuscular injections and can be given prior to surgery, *neoadjuvant*, or after surgery, *adjuvant*. The primary role of systemic therapy is to find and then remove cancer cells that have escaped the breast. One ongoing issue for breast cancer doctors is that we don't have accurate, predictable tests to tell us if any cancer cells have traveled elsewhere in the body. I think we are getting closer to finding just such a test, but until that time we must continue treating all women with systemic therapy whom we suspect may need it. More about how we decide whether you might benefit from systemic treatment will be discussed later in this chapter.

Over the last forty years, clinical research trials have proved that the use of systemic therapy combined with local control (surgery) increases the cure rate of women with breast cancer. This systemic therapy *after* local treatment is called *adjuvant* systemic therapy. Adjuvant means "added on." Later in the manual I will address adjuvant and neoadjuvant systemic therapy for each of the four breast cancer types described in chapter 3 in more detail. I have divided the therapies into three categories: hormonal, chemotherapies (what we call cytotoxic agents or cell poisons), and *others*, which are exciting new agents that target specific mutations in the cancer cell.

Hormone Therapy

❧ Approximately 70 percent of invasive breast cancers have hormone receptors on the surface of the cancer cells. As discussed in chapter 3, we call these *Luminal* breast cancers. These cancers are influenced by the hormone estrogen and/or progesterone. With more than forty years of research and clinical trials, we know that blocking the receptor or preventing the cell from receiving estrogen via the receptor can make the cancer cell die.

One of the first clinical trials, the NSABP-B14 trial, was conducted more than thirty-five years ago and treated 2,644 women with estrogen-receptor-positive, lymph-node-negative, surgically removed breast cancer with either an oral drug called tamoxifen or a placebo pill for five years. Tamoxifen is an estrogen-like drug that strongly binds to the estrogen receptor on the surface of the cancer cell, preventing *true* estrogen from stimulating and promoting the cancer cell to grow and divide. Tamoxifen is one of a class of drugs called a _selective estrogen receptor modulator_ (SERM). The NSABP-B14 trial was a huge success: the women receiving tamoxifen had about a 30 percent decrease in systemic relapse compared to the placebo group. The tamoxifen group also had significantly fewer local recurrences and second breast cancers. A five-year course of tamoxifen became the standard treatment for women with estrogen-receptor-positive breast cancer.

Various other trials have built upon the NSABP-B14. In the late 1980s, the Stockholm trial compared taking two years of tamoxifen versus five years and found the longer duration was more effective. The NSABP-B14 trial had some patients in the tamoxifen group continue taking the pill beyond five years. Early analysis at year seven seemed to suggest that continuing the tamoxifen for longer than five years was not beneficial, so the trial ended. More recently, however, two large trials to compare five years versus ten years of taking tamoxifen were conducted in Europe (the ATLAS and the ATTOM trials), and both demonstrated a small, relapse-free survival advantage in those women who continued for ten years. Does this mean that your oncologist will prescribe tamoxifen for ten years? Probably not, because a recent genomic test, known as the Breast Cancer Index (BCI), has been developed to determine the benefit of endocrine therapy.

For more than twenty years, taking adjuvant tamoxifen for five years following surgery, with or without chemotherapy, was the standard treatment for women with Luminal breast cancer. It was well tolerated with rare but serious side effects of venous blood clots and endometrial (uterine) cancer. I would guess that I have given around ten thousand women tamoxifen in my career, and I have had no fatality from either of these side effects; in fact, close to a thousand women have been cured because of the drug.

A new class of hormone treatment was developed in the late 1990s known as the aromatase inhibitors (AIs). In contrast to premenopausal women, whose estrogen is produced mostly in the ovaries, postmenopausal women's estrogen is mainly produced by the adrenal gland and peripheral tissues. It was discovered that estrogen production in these women could be greatly reduced by inhibiting the aromatase enzyme that was necessary for the final conversion of androstenedione to estrogen. Tamoxifen remained the treatment for premenopausal women, but the AIs offered an alternative treatment by greatly reducing available estrogen necessary for the hormone-dependent cancer's survival. Figure 6.1 diagrams the different mechanism of action of tamoxifen and the AIs.

A large clinical trial, the ATAC trial, compared adjuvant tamoxifen to anastrozole (Arimidex) for five years in postmenopausal women following local control. Anastrozole was slightly better in preventing recurrence, but now, after twenty years, there is no overall difference in survival between the two groups.

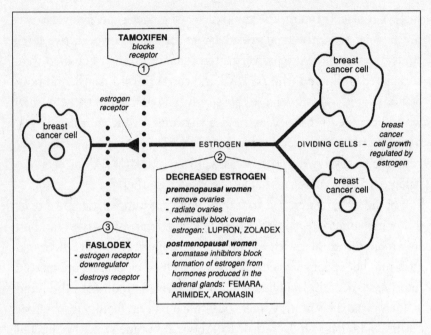

Figure 6.1

Regulating estrogen exposure to affect breast cancer cell growth

There are three different AIs: anastrozole (Arimidex) and letrozole (Femara), which are nonsteroidal inhibitors of the enzyme aromatase, and exemestane (Aromasin), which is a steroidal inhibitor. All three appear to be equivalent in preventing recurrence. The AIs have different side effects than tamoxifen—no stimulation of the uterine lining or venous blood clots, but there is increased bone loss, and women complain of achiness and stiffness in their joints. (See Table 6.1 on the side effects of AIs and tamoxifen.)

AI for a total of five years gave the same results as five years of tamoxifen. My own experience is that postmenopausal women tolerate tamoxifen better than an AI from a quality-of-life perspective, so I usually start with tamoxifen and switch to an AI after a few years.

Hormonal therapy is now being offered to women before breast cancer surgery (neoadjuvant) for three to twelve months with resulting

Side Effects	Tamoxifen	Aromatase Inhibitor
Hot flashes	---	++
Bone loss	---	+++
Uterine thickening	+ (10% of cases)	---
Joint and bone achiness	+	+++
Venous blood clots	+ (<5% of cases)	---
Weight gain	+	+
Vaginal thinning	+/---	++

Table 6.1

Common side effects of hormonal therapy

Smith IE. N Engl J Med 2003; 348: 243–244

regression of the cancer. This approach has been much more prevalent in Europe than in the United States, but it is now more widely done worldwide. It allows for more women to have WLE rather than mastectomy and for more flexibility around the timing of the surgery. Clinical trials are looking to see if adding additional treatments to hormonal therapy prior to breast surgery can lead to an even better response. We will discuss hormonal therapy in more detail in chapter 8 when we discuss the treatment of the *Luminal* subtype of breast cancer.

Unfortunately, in spite of five to ten years of adjuvant hormonal therapy, some women will develop resistance and recur systemically. This "hormonal resistance" has become a major area of breast cancer research. With the recent ability of scientists to sequence the genes in the cancer cell, mutations have been discovered that appear to be responsible for resistance to AIs and tamoxifen. New drugs are being developed based on these mutations. Two drugs, everolimus (Afinitor) and palbociclib (Ibrance), have been approved for use in women that have relapsed and are being tested in clinical trials in the adjuvant setting, and there are a number of other promising agents under investigation.

Chemotherapy

_✁_ Chemotherapy is certainly the most feared and dreaded part of breast cancer treatment. The good news is that we have made tremendous progress in the last thirty years in drug development, correct dosing, and preventing, managing, or eliminating side effects.

The goal of chemotherapy is to eradicate cancer cells that have spread from the primary breast cancer into the bloodstream to the rest of the body. In the 1980s and 1990s, a majority of women with invasive breast cancers larger than one centimeter (½ inch) or with spread to an axillary (underarm) lymph node were prescribed chemotherapy. In 2018, we are now able to better select those women that will benefit from chemotherapy based on the characteristics of the cancer and using new genomic tools that analyze the cancer for genes that are responsible for spread. We give much less chemotherapy today than we have in the past, and the regimens we use are far more effective.

What we need is a test that accurately detects evidence of spread into the system, a test that can determine who requires chemotherapy and who can be cured with local control alone. A huge amount of research on this subject is under way, and I believe we are on the verge of developing such a test. My prediction is that it will involve the ability to detect a tumor-specific protein or DNA fragment of tumor origin present in the blood after the primary cancer is removed. Hopefully by the next edition of this manual we will have a result to share with readers. Table 6.2 lists factors that your oncologist will consider and use to make decisions.

Chemotherapy works because it affects dividing cells. The more rapidly a cancer cell goes through cell division—what we call mitosis— the greater the killing effect of the chemotherapy. Cancer cells are much more vulnerable to chemotherapy than noncancerous cells because they are more "fragile." Yes, fragile. They lack the ability to repair DNA damage (unlike normal cells with DNA repair genes), and cancer cells are constantly going through cell division. Figure 6.2 is a

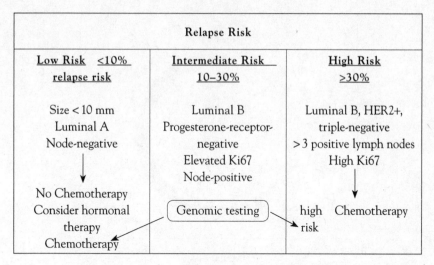

Relapse Risk		
Low Risk **<10%** **relapse risk**	**Intermediate Risk** **10–30%**	**High Risk** **>30%**
Size < 10 mm Luminal A Node-negative ↓ No Chemotherapy Consider hormonal therapy Chemotherapy	Luminal B Progesterone-receptor- negative Elevated Ki67 Node-positive Genomic testing	Luminal B, HER2+, triple-negative > 3 positive lymph nodes High Ki67 ↓ high Chemotherapy risk

Table 6.2

Decision factors for chemotherapy

depiction of the cell cycle. Most normal cells go through the cell cycle with the exception of brain and heart muscle cells. Chemotherapy will have little effect on normal cells that are resting in the G1 part of the cycle and infrequently enter the S phase duplicating DNA. As you can see, cancer cells that are frequently and regularly passing through G2 and mitosis will be quite vulnerable to the cytotoxic effects of chemotherapy.

Chemotherapy drugs affect different sites of DNA replication and division. Protocols have been developed that combine several drugs together with different sites of action that give additive and synergistic killing effects. Chemotherapy drugs can be linked to agents such as antibodies that directly target the cancer cell, sparing normal cells. We will discuss specific regimens of chemotherapy in the following chapters that address the treatment of the breast cancer subtypes. Chemotherapy regimens have been developed over the last few decades through multiple clinical trials comparing various types, dosage schedules, and combinations of drugs. Chemotherapy can be given before removing the primary cancer. We call this "preoperative "or "neoadjuvant"

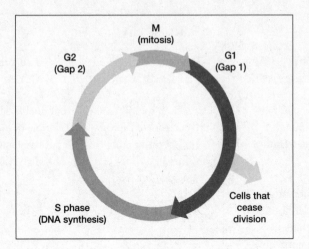

Figure 6.2
The cell cycle

chemotherapy. Alternatively, chemotherapy can be administered after surgery. This sequence is called "adjuvant." Adjuvant means "added on."

The chemotherapy drug regimen is given intravenously and then there is a recovery period for the normal cells to recover. Each administration and recovery period is called a "cycle." Each cycle is one to three weeks depending on the drugs and dosages. Neoadjuvant or adjuvant chemotherapy is usually given over a period of twelve to eighteen weeks.

Neoadjuvant Chemotherapy

In recent years there has been a movement in breast cancer treatment to give systemic treatment prior to surgery—what we call neoadjuvant. This has become possible because modern tumor imaging and needle biopsies provide all the information about the cancer that is available before surgery—information that once required removal of the primary cancer and regional lymph nodes. After obtaining this information, if the risk of systemic spread is deemed sufficient to require chemotherapy, there are some advantages to giving the chemotherapy prior to surgery:

1. Chemotherapy will affect the primary breast cancer and involved lymph nodes and will frequently downsize or in some cases completely eradicate the cancer. This means less surgery with fewer lymph nodes that need to be removed, and may be associated with a better cosmetic result, too.
2. It's helpful for your doctors to know if the chemotherapy is working (or, rarely, is not working) before surgery.
3. Chemotherapy can be given earlier, without the necessary delay for recovery from surgery.
4. There is important prognostic information obtained by the extent of response to the chemotherapy. Often at the time of surgery no cancer can be detected in the breast and lymph nodes during physical exam or by imaging (this represents a *clinical* complete response) and no invasive cancer can be seen by the pathologist under a microscope (a *pathologic* complete response, or pCR). There is a high correlation between a "cure" and a pCR in certain cancers, like the triple-negative type. If chemotherapy is given after surgery (adjuvant), the ability to measure the response is lost.
5. If there is no response or a partial response after the first few treatments (which occurs in less than 10 percent of cases in our experience), the removed cancer can then be studied after surgery, so postsurgery treatment can be better selected if deemed necessary.

In the past, there has often been a rush to remove the cancer—on the part of the patient and the surgeon. This is understandable in that no one wants a potentially dangerous cancer to remain in their body. My experience over many years is that women "want the cancer out *now*." This is changing and, once educated, women are willing to consider neoadjuvant therapy if indicated. I would certainly discuss this with your surgeon oncologist. And patients report how relieving it is to watch and feel the cancer shrinking.

Toxicity from Chemotherapy

✂ Chemotherapy is toxic and has side effects. With improved anti-nausea medications, however, the once severe side effects of nausea and vomiting have been essentially eliminated and are rarely a problem. Many drugs used in breast cancer patients do still affect the hair follicles, and temporary hair loss is common (see Figure 6.3). During the few hours following the administration of the chemo, the hair protein that is made in the follicle is damaged, and when it gets to the surface about two weeks later, the hair will break off at that point. Many centers are beginning to offer scalp cooling devices during drug administration, which prevents damage to the protein. It is moderately uncomfortable and prolongs the chemo administration time, but is

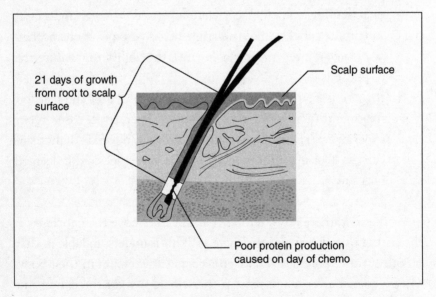

Figure 6.3
Hair follicle

about 80 percent effective (depending on the chemotherapy regimen). This is something you may want to discuss with your oncologist.

Fatigue is a very common complaint and tends to afflict patients early in each treatment cycle. Patients generally recover before the next cycle begins but have some cumulative effect over the entire course of treatment. Fortunately, once the chemotherapy is complete, there is usually full recovery within four to six weeks.

Some of the drugs, particularly the taxanes (paclitaxel and docetaxel) and Carboplatinum, can cause neuropathy, which usually manifests as numbness and tingling of the distal extremities (fingers and toes) and, in some cases, alteration of taste. Neuropathy is usually mild and reversible, but the reversal can take a few months.

For younger, premenopausal women, chemotherapy can affect the ovaries and can cause premature ovarian failure and infertility. The risk of this depends on the age of the woman and the chemotherapy regimen prescribed. There are ways to protect the ovaries using medications that block ovarian-stimulating hormones from the pituitary. This should be discussed with your oncologist. Fertility is a major concern for some younger women. Even with ovarian suppression during chemotherapy, a majority of women under forty will recover ovarian function. The eggs in the ovary do not seem to be damaged by the chemotherapy since they are "resting" and not dividing. Egg harvesting is an option prior to starting chemotherapy and is quite successful with newer techniques. If this an issue for you, you will want to see a fertility specialist. For the women with hormone-positive (usually Luminal B) breast cancer, hormone therapy, usually tamoxifen, is prescribed after chemotherapy for a minimum of five years. This will further delay pregnancy because tamoxifen interferes with ovulation, and with pregnancy it may cause fetal harm.

The most serious risk during chemotherapy is infection. As discussed earlier in the chapter, the drugs affect rapidly dividing cells. Some of the most rapidly dividing cells are in the bone marrow, including the white blood cells that fight bacterial infections called granulocytes. Chemotherapy can temporarily reduce granulocyte levels, which leads to an increased risk of potentially serious infection. If the chemotherapy regimen is associated with a significant decrease in granulocyte production, your oncologist will administer a "growth factor" to stimulate the bone marrow to recover more rapidly after each chemotherapy. Platelets that prevent bleeding are also produced in the bone marrow and can be affected by some chemotherapy regimens (usually less than the granulocyte production). Your oncologist will monitor your blood counts carefully and determine if you need reductions in dosage or "growth factor" support.

The issue of mental or cognitive dysfunction resulting from chemotherapy is a topic much discussed in support groups and on the Internet. This issue is complex because it involves a number of factors: effects of chemotherapy on the ovaries and decreased hormone levels, stress, drugs used for sedation, nausea, anxiety, and sleep. The term *chemonesia* has emerged to describe this mental dysfunction. I believe this side effect is temporary and is reversible. A vast majority of women receiving adjuvant or neoadjuvant chemotherapy are able to return to and maintain their normal quality of life once treatment is done with no residual effects.

One chemotherapy drug we use in certain treatment plans can cause two rare but serious side effects. The drug, doxorubicin (Adriamycin),

Hormonal	Chemotherapy	Antibodies

A. SERMs
   Tamoxifen
   Toremifeme (Fareston)
B. Aromatase Inhibitors
   Anastrozole (Arimidex)
   Letrozole (Femara)
   Exemestane (Aromasin)
C. Ovarian Suppression
   Lupron
   Zoladex
	Doxorubicin
	Cyclophosphamide
	Fluorouracil
	Capecitabine (Xeloda)
	Carboplatinum
	Docetaxel (Taxotere)
	Paclitaxel (Taxol)
		Trastuzumab (Herceptin)
		Pertuzumab (Perjeta)

Table 6.3

Common adjuvant and neoadjuvant systemic therapies for breast cancer can cause heart damage and acute leukemia in a very small percentage of patients. If your oncologist is recommending this drug, he or she will need to discuss these risks with you.

Table 6.3 lists the most common systemic therapies and related compounds used in adjuvant and neoadjuvant regimens today. We will discuss the treatment of each breast cancer subtype and the regimens used specifically for each subtype in the following three chapters, along with promising systemic therapies that are in clinical trials and close to FDA approval.

7

. . . . . .

❧

Ductal Carcinoma in Situ

This chapter is written specifically for women with ductal carcinoma in situ (DCIS). If you have invasive breast cancer, you will probably want to skip this chapter and move on to chapter 8. Because of the increasing incidence of DCIS, which accounts for about 20 percent of newly diagnosed breast cancer, and the controversies and complexities in management, it is necessary to devote an entire chapter to this topic. More cases of DCIS have been identified in recent years through the increased use of screening mammography. Once it was discovered that clusters of unique calcifications in the breast represented preinvasive, nonpalpable cancer, we could diagnose cancer from a mammogram before it went on to become invasive.

The good news with this early form of breast cancer is that it is completely curable with local control because it has not had a chance to spread to lymph and blood vessels. The challenge has been the development of appropriate treatment options to achieve local control. Early attempts at surgeries that were less than mastectomies often fail when surgical margins were inadequate, leaving microscopic residual cancer behind. To counter this, radiation therapy was added to partial mastectomy and did seem to increase the local control rate. However, the effects of radiation on tissues reduced desired cosmetic outcome over time, and for those patients who did have a recurrence or a second event (although rare), mastectomy with reconstruction was compromised by the radiation effects on the tissues.

Our past experience in treating DCIS indicates that breast conservation is feasible and successful when the area of involvement is small in size, the surgical margins free of disease around the cancer are large, and the cancer cells are low-grade. In this type of DCIS radiation adds little benefit. For larger DCIS, mastectomy has become much more accepted because of the excellent advances in reconstruction that are often capable of sparing skin and even nipples (if DCIS is adequately separated from the nipple). For DCIS where wide local excision (WLE) is an option but there is an increased risk of recurrence due to close margins or high microscopic grade, the addition of radiation lowers the recurrence rate.

What are the numbers? Mastectomy is 100 percent successful in curing this preinvasive breast cancer. In low-risk disease, WLE without radiation has a success rate of about 90 percent (1 percent per year recurrence over ten years). For women with higher-risk DCIS, WLE is approximately 75 percent successful without radiation. If radiation is added, the success rate approaches 90 percent. We will discuss criteria for radiation use in high-risk DCIS later in the chapter.

If there is a recurrence with WLE, it remains DCIS about 50 percent of the time. In the other 50 percent of instances it will become invasive. The good news is that survival, regardless of the treatment, is the same, approximately 100 percent. This is because women with WLE treatment are followed carefully with annual mammograms. Local recurrences are almost always detected on a surveillance mammogram at the early stages and treated successfully without systemic relapse.

As discussed in chapter 1, DCIS is a ductal cancer that has not penetrated the basement membrane separating the milk duct from the underlying breast tissue that contains blood and lymph vessels (see Figure 1.2 in chapter 1). If the cancer is found at this stage, there is no risk of its spreading into the blood or lymphatic system, and the risk of dying from breast cancer is essentially zero. Fortunately, DCIS is relatively

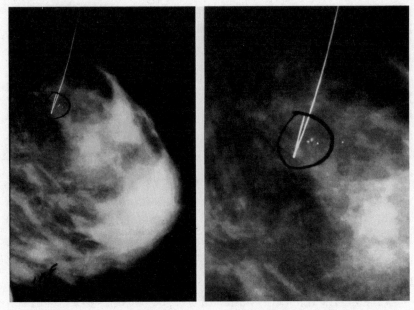

Small cluster of calcification
(low-grade DCIS)

Magnified view with hook and wire

Figure 7.1

Mammogram with calcifications

easy to detect before invasion occurs. On the mammogram, DCIS appears as a speckling of calcifications or as a change in the breast structure that has a very characteristic appearance to the radiologist (Figure 7.1). The calcifications are dead cancer cells that have petrified (*calcified*) inside the ducts. These *flecks* of calcium have nothing to do with dietary calcium intake. Like invasive breast cancer, DCIS is a *heterogeneous* (variable) disease. According to the medical literature, a majority of these cancers will become invasive if left untreated or undiscovered. The cell that becomes cancerous can vary in aggressiveness and growth rate. Some forms of DCIS are low-grade and very slow-growing. Under the microscope, the cells are fairly small and resemble normal breast ductal cells.

This form of DCIS is often associated with calcifications that have a powdery appearance on the mammogram. Under the micro-

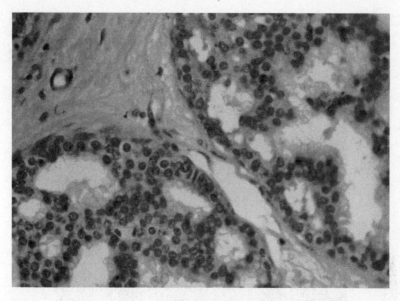

Figure 7.2
Small cell DCIS without necrosis

scope, there is little evidence of *necrosis* (dead cellular material) in the center of the ducts (Figure 7.2). Because of the absence of *necrotic* material, known as *comedo necrosis*, this type of DCIS is termed *non-comedo.*

At the other end of the DCIS spectrum is the high-grade form, which is fast-growing with many cells dividing. Cancer cells in the center of the duct die, resulting in calcifications that look like branching tree limbs on a mammogram (Figure 7.3) and prominent areas of *central duct necrosis* under the microscope. (Figure 7.4). If this type of DCIS, termed *comedo*, is allowed to grow and become invasive, it is potentially very dangerous because of its rapid growth rate. There are also intermediate forms of DCIS that fall between the two ends of the spectrum.

The challenge in treating DCIS is to remove the cancer completely from the breast. Surgical excision of the DCIS, along with a clear surrounding *margin* of normal breast tissue, is the primary treatment. The margin of uninvolved breast tissue is important in preventing a

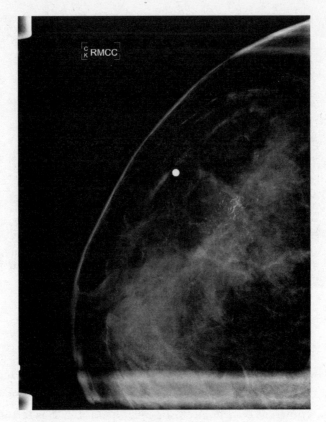

Figure 7.3
Branching calcifications of high-grade DCIS

recurrence from cancer cells that could be left behind following surgery. Ideally, the breast surgeon must remove the cancerous tissue and leave at least a two-millimeter *clear margin* (normal tissue) but a ten-millimeter clear margin is ideal. This can be difficult if the area of DCIS involvement is large or is close to the skin or chest wall. The extra ten-millimeter margin that the surgeon attempts to remove in these cases can substantially increase the size of the tissue removed and leave the patient with a deformity or a much smaller breast.

The radiologist can greatly assist the surgeon in planning the best surgical approach possible. Advances in breast MRI have been very helpful to the surgeon, particularly for locating high-grade DCIS. In

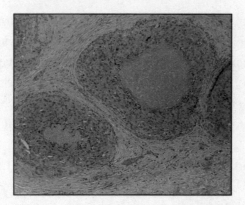

Figure 7.4
DCIS high-grade *comedo* type

most cases there is no palpable lump with DCIS; therefore, the radiologist must assist the surgeon by placing markers, usually in the form of multiple wire hooks, where the cancer appears in the breast tissue. This guides the surgeon in the operating room to know exactly what portion of breast tissue must be removed.

Breast surgeons learned from early experience that if the area of DCIS was small and they cleared wide margins with an *excisional biopsy*, the cancer would not recur in most women. For larger areas of involvement, it was often impossible for surgeons to clear the margins adequately to prevent recurrence yet leave the breast with an acceptable size and symmetry. In these latter cases, most women chose simple mastectomy, often with immediate reconstruction, resulting in a cure rate of close to a hundred percent.

Clinical trials have demonstrated that the combination of radiation and surgery reduces the recurrence rates when the cancer's involvement is large and the margins are close. Radiation, however, is less effective when DCIS is high-grade and large and when there are close margins. Additional clinical trials have revealed that the drug tamoxifen further reduces recurrence rates and also prevents the development of new cancers in the opposite breast. This drug is only effective in patients whose DCIS is *estrogen-receptor-positive*.

Flow diagram 7.1 demonstrates how we manage treatment of DCIS at Breastlink. There are two fundamental treatment decisions to be made in the management of ductal carcinoma in situ. First, is mastectomy required, or can an acceptable local control rate be achieved with less than mastectomy (WLE) and with an acceptable cosmetic result? Second, if a wide local excision (WLE) is possible, should radiation be added to increase the local control rate?

Four randomized trials have demonstrated that the addition of radiation to WLE reduces local recurrence by approximately 15 percent. Put another way, women in the trials who were given no radiation had a local control of 75 percent, and those given radiation had a 90 percent control rate. Based on these trials, radiation will be recommended to a majority of women who chose less than a mastectomy for treatment of their DCIS. But 75 percent of women will receive no benefit from radiation and could be cured with surgery alone. Another 10 percent of women will experience recurrence despite receiving radiation, leaving the 15 percent who benefit.

The challenge for us is to determine which women can be spared radiation. We know low-risk women have small areas of involvement and low-grade characteristics of cancer cells visible under the microscope, so if the surgeon can achieve clear margins of five to ten millimeters, then the chance of recurrence is decreased to 10 percent. Researchers have created scoring systems based on the size, margins, and grade of cancer and the age of the patient, but a majority of women with DCIS will have one or more characteristics that are borderline, making such systems imperfect.

At the time of surgery for DCIS, the microscopic evaluation of the DCIS rarely reveals very early invasion (called *microinvasion*). Research and experience has revealed that this does not affect outcome or change treatment as long as the microinvasion is small.

I must admit we tend to overtreat, and that's why radiation in recent years has become a part of most treatment plans for women with DCIS not treated by mastectomy. As difficult as a local recurrence is psychologically, with careful surveillance there is minimal

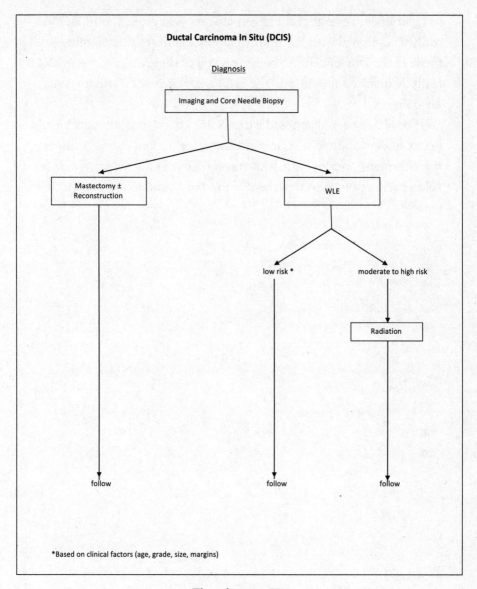

Flow diagram 7.1
Management of DCIS

risk of systemic relapse, even though some of these recurrences are invasive.

Researchers are developing genomic assays of the DCIS specimens looking for activated genes that might predict aggressiveness and risk of recurrence. Several of these genomic tools appear promising, especially if combined with the traditional risk factors of size, margins, and grade of the cancer cell. Although several of these assays are commercially available, it is early and the utility of these tests is still unclear in my opinion.

If you have been diagnosed with DCIS, I hope that you now have a better understanding of your cancer and feel more confident discussing treatment options with your surgeon. You and your team can develop your personalized treatment plan from a combination of effective options.

8
. . . . . .

૪

Management of Luminal Breast Cancer

In chapter 3 we defined Luminal breast cancer as the breast cancer cell type that has receptors for estrogen and progesterone on the cell surface but no HER2 receptors. This type of breast cancer accounts for approximately 70 percent of newly diagnosed invasive breast cancers. Luminal breast cancer has two fairly distinct subtypes: Luminal A and Luminal B. This division is important because the two subtypes differ in prognosis, risk of recurrence, and optimal treatment options.

To determine if you have Luminal A or Luminal B, your doctor will rely on a number of factors that include appearance of cancer cells under the microscope and special immunohistochemical (IHC) stains that measure the amount of hormone receptors on the cancer-cell surface and detect the absence of the HER2-type receptor. A special IHC stain, the Ki67 stain, measures the percentage of cells entering cell division (mitosis) and is also very important. In difficult cases your doctor may resort to genomic testing to sort out the subtype. Table 8.1 summarizes the characteristics that help define Luminal A versus Luminal B breast cancer.

Luminal A cancers tend to be slow-growing and strongly hormone-receptor-positive, and they infrequently spread outside the breast. Luminal B cancers are more aggressive and grow more rapidly. Under a

Characteristics	Luminal A	Luminal B
Estrogen receptor	Strongly positive	Strong to weakly positive
Progesterone receptor	Strongly positive	Weak to absent
Tumor grade (MBR)	Low	Moderate to high
Ki67	Low	Moderate to high
Lymph nodes	Usually negative	Negative to positive
Genomic testing	Low-risk	Intermediate- to high-risk

Table 8.1

Luminal A and B characteristics

microscope, more cells in Luminal B cancers are seen dividing, which is reflected by an increased Ki67 staining. There are often fewer hormone receptors or even a total lack of progesterone receptors on the cell surface of Luminal B cancer cells. Luminal B cancers tend to be found in younger women and are more likely than Luminal A cancers to have lymph node spread. We will now discuss management of each subtype.

Luminal A Breast Cancer

✎ Luminal A subtype accounts for about 40 to 50 percent of all invasive breast cancers. This is a slow-growing breast cancer and is most often discovered on a screening mammogram. It is more common in older women, but it can affect younger premenopausal women when it presents as a slow-growing, palpable lump, often confused with a cyst or fibroadenoma. Diagnosis is usually made by a needle biopsy. All the information to make the proper diagnosis can be obtained from the needle biopsy and breast imaging (mammograms, ultrasounds, and sometimes MRI) to develop a treatment plan.

Treatment involves primarily local control by surgery. A majority of women will have no spread to the axillary lymph nodes, but this is usually determined by removal of the sentinel node (chapter 5). Radiation is usually prescribed for women under age sixty-five or seventy who choose partial mastectomy or wide local excision (WLE). As discussed in chapter 5, this can be intraoperative radiation at the time of surgery or partial breast radiation. Flow diagram 8.1 describes how we manage Luminal A breast cancer at Breastlink.

The prognosis for women with Luminal A breast cancer who receive local control treatment is excellent, with a cure rate that exceeds 90 percent. However, there is a survival benefit to adding systemic hormonal therapy after surgery and radiation. Unfortunately, we don't know who actually needs the adjuvant hormonal treatment, and so the standard of care is to offer hormonal therapy to most women with Luminal A breast cancer. The good news is that Luminal A breast cancers do not benefit from or need cytotoxic chemotherapy.

Is there a way to identify women diagnosed with Luminal A cancer who will not benefit from hormonal therapy and who can be cured with local control alone? While over 80 percent of Luminal A breast cancers are cured by surgery, we treat most of these women with a minimum of five years of hormonal therapy, too, using either tamoxifen or an aromatase inhibitor (AI). Certainly these treatments are less toxic than chemotherapy, but there are still side effects, and the length of treatment is substantial. With this in mind, researchers are looking for tools that will allow us to predict who will benefit from hormonal treatment.

A further promising approach may be to monitor the disappearance of circulating-tumor DNA following surgery. The hypothesis here is that localized cancer in the breast is shedding DNA fragments into the blood that we can measure because of their unique cancer mutations. If the DNA fragments disappear after surgery and do not reappear within six months, this might indicate that there is no spread of cancer into the bloodstream and out into the body so five years of hormonal therapy can be avoided. What needs to be determined is whether

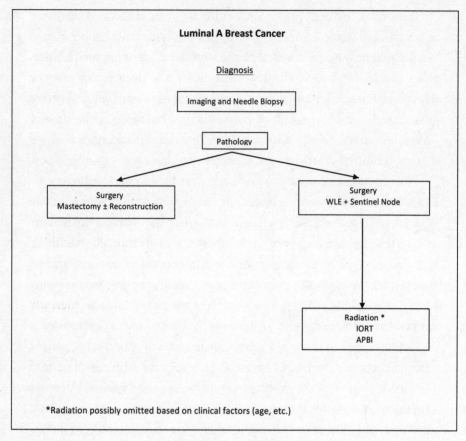

Flow diagram 8.1

Management of Luminal A breast cancer

Luminal A cancers consistently shed mutated DNA fragments into the blood that can be detected. At the time of publication of this sixth edition, this test is close to becoming commercially available. A number of companies are currently measuring and tracking circulating-tumor DNA.

Another possibility is a genomic analysis of the cancer that is predictive of benefit from hormonal therapy. We already have this type of genomic testing that predicts benefit of chemotherapy in Luminal B cancers.

In the 1980s, after the development of tamoxifen, a number of re-search trials were conducted to determine if giving tamoxifen to women with Luminal breast cancer would prevent systemic recurrence. Researchers conducted a study in the United States, known as the NSABP-B14 trial, which compared women with early Luminal breast cancer who were given either tamoxifen or a placebo for five years. Results indicated that the women who received tamoxifen had about a relative 35 percent increase in survival versus the placebo group, 91 percent versus 85 percent disease-free survival at ten years.

A similar study was conducted in Sweden, known as the Stockholm trial (Figure 8.2). Six hundred postmenopausal women with early Luminal breast cancer were given tamoxifen or placebo. The study par-ticipants received two years of tamoxifen. Half of three hundred women went on to receive tamoxifen for another three more years, or a total of five years. Results of this study showed that five years of tamoxifen was more effective than two years in preventing recurrence. The tumors of the six hundred women were preserved, and we have long-term (greater than twenty years) survival data on the entire study group. The trial confirmed the efficacy of taking tamoxifen and demonstrated that five years was better than two years. The interesting thing to me is that recently a biotech company, Biotheranostics, has developed a seven-gene tumor assay called the Breast Cancer Index (BCI). They obtained the tumor tissue from the six hundred participants in the Stockholm trial and applied the seven-gene test to tissue samples. Two of the genes, HoxB13 (H) and IL17BR (I), are estrogen-signaling genes. Women who had a low ratio of the H/I genes had an extremely low relapse rate twenty years into remission, and for these women taking tamoxifen rather than a placebo made no difference in relapse-free survival.

More recently, another biotech company called Agendia completed a similar study, also using stored tumor tissue from the Stockholm trial, but utilizing a seventy-gene assay. Agendia found that women with a very low (or *ultra low*) score on their MammaPrint test had excellent long-term survival rates regardless of whether they received tamoxifen or a placebo.

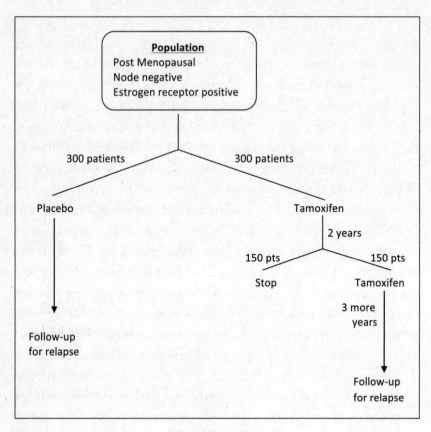

Flow diagram 8.2
Stockholm trial

My conclusion is that in the near future, using new technologies such as circulating tumor DNA or genomic testing like the BCI, we will be able to identify those women with Luminal A breast cancer who will be cured with surgery alone, sparing them five years of hormonal therapy. I need to mention that there are secondary benefits to being on hormonal therapy. Women receiving tamoxifen or AIs to prevent systemic recurrence also benefit by having a reduced risk of another unrelated breast cancer.

Length of Hormonal Treatment

✳ As discussed in chapter 6, the Stockholm trial demonstrated that there is a survival benefit from tamoxifen treatment and that five years of treatment was more effective than two years, but the NSABP-B14 trial extended tamoxifen beyond five years and showed no improvement. However, it is now thought this was a premature conclusion and that if the trial had been allowed to continue for the full ten years, there may have been a benefit for ten years over five years. More recently, two large trials for women with Luminal breast cancer, ATLAS and ATTOM, have shown a survival benefit for patients receiving tamoxifen for ten years over five years.

At this time, after reviewing the literature, my personal conclusion is that five years of tamoxifen or an AI is probably sufficient treatment for Luminal A breast cancer. However, this may not be true for Luminal B cancers. The BCI test has been validated to predict the subset of women who will benefit from extended hormonal treatment. A small fragment of the preserved cancer can be requested and sent to Biotheranostics for analysis, and they will provide a score that tells you the risk that the cancer will recur after five years of remission and the likelihood that extended hormonal treatment will be beneficial.

Type of Hormonal Therapy: Tamoxifen Versus Aromatase Inhibitor

✳ As I mentioned in chapter 6, there are two types of hormonal therapy that lower estrogen levels in the body, since estrogen is necessary for the cancer to survive. The first, tamoxifen, is a *selective estrogen receptor modulator* (SERM), which is an estrogen-like molecule that blocks the estrogen receptor on the cancer cell membrane. It has a very strong affinity for the estrogen receptor and works when endogenous estrogen is present, so it is effective in premenopausal women who still have ovarian function.

Next are the three aromatase inhibitors that act to inhibit estrogen production mainly in the adrenal gland but also in other tissues. They prevent the conversion of androstenedione to estrogen, causing extremely low levels of estrogen in the body.

For cases of Luminal A breast cancer, tamoxifen is the preferred option for younger premenopausal women. For postmenopausal patients, both tamoxifen and AIs are effective. They have different mechanisms of action (Figure 6.1) and different toxicity and side effect profiles (Table 6.1).

Several large studies have compared tamoxifen to AIs. The ATAC trial compared tamoxifen to arimidex, as well as to a combination of both. The BIG I-198 trial compared tamoxifen to the AI, to letrozole, and to a sequence of tamoxifen for two years followed by letrozole for three years. They also tested the reverse order—letrozole followed by tamoxifen. In both studies the AIs seemed to be *slightly* superior to tamoxifen, but my interpretation is that in Luminal A tumors the options were fairly equal in preventing recurrence, and overall survival at twenty years is essentially the same. Interestingly, the sequential doses of tamoxifen followed by letrozole yielded results equivalent to those after five years of just letrozole—this for both the Luminal A and B groups.

One must then weigh the side effects of the two types of treatment. Initially, when the AIs were introduced by the pharmaceutical industry, they were promoted as safer and better tolerated than tamoxifen. Tamoxifen, as an estrogen derivative, can promote uterine hyperplasia in a small percentage of women, which can lead to uterus (endometrial) cancer. Because of its estrogen activity, tamoxifen can also cause venous blood clots in susceptible women. Both side effects are rare but potentially dangerous.

The AIs can cause accelerated bone loss leading to osteoporosis, but there are medications that can neutralize the loss of bone. Clinical trials demonstrated that the AIs—anastrozole, letrozole, and exemestane—were equivalent to and a safer alternative to tamoxifen. However, side effects from the AIs began to emerge. Women began to complain of body aches and stiffness—not all women, but a significant number, many of whom stopped taking the medication. Apparently, the small amount of adrenal estrogen is important to their sense of well-being. In my practice, postmenopausal women with Luminal A cancer and an excellent chance of cure frequently decided to stop the AI and were willing to sacrifice a small survival advantage for better quality of life. In our practice, we ask women to switch to tamoxifen rather than stop treatment, and many have found it to be more tolerable.

One of the side effects of menopause is vaginal thinning (atrophy) and dryness. An advantage of tamoxifen is that it is safe to prescribe vaginal estrogen to counter this. Oncologists are concerned that women taking AIs may absorb enough estrogen transvaginally to overcome the blockade created by the AI.

Some menopausal symptoms appear in women taking either tamoxifen or the aromatase inhibitors. They tend to be more pronounced in women who recently entered menopause or stopped taking hormone replacement therapy. Fortunately, these symptoms of flushing (hot flashes), insomnia, achiness, and others are transient and get better over time. But for some women, the symptoms are uncomfortable or disturbing enough for them to consider stopping treatment. It is important for you to discuss this with your oncologist. There are some herbs and homeopathic aids that appear safe and can help relieve these symptoms.

Preoperative Hormonal Treatment

❦ There has been a movement to treat breast cancer patients who have high-grade (fast-growing) cancers with chemotherapy before surgery. These are *not* Luminal A cancers but high-grade Luminal B, HER2-positive, and triple-negative breast cancers. We will discuss this thoroughly in the following chapters. But the same principles that apply to treating Luminal A and some Luminal B breast cancers with estrogen-targeted therapy before surgery apply here. The advantages are the following:

1. The cancer will reduce in size and make surgery less deforming.
2. There will be measurable and visible proof that the hormonal treatment is working.
3. The surgery can be done in a nonemergent and convenient time frame.
4. Many women are able to have breast-conserving surgery rather than a mastectomy.

Most of the use of preoperative hormonal therapy has been in post-menopausal women. Interestingly, the use of preoperative estrogen-targeted therapy is very common in Europe, where up to 40 percent of women with Luminal breast cancer receive preoperative tamoxifen or AI therapy for up to six months. For reasons that are unclear, U.S. oncologists rarely prescribe preoperative or neoadjuvant estrogen-directed treatment. Because of the merits of this approach, I believe this will change in the future, and in fact the subject is frequently addressed at national breast cancer conferences now. The length of time for treatment is longer than the preoperative chemotherapy protocols and is usually in the range of six months, but we have been using this approach successfully in Breastlink clinics. It requires careful monitoring, and the patient must have a good understanding of the approach and feel comfortable with delaying surgery.

Lymph Node Involvement in Luminal A Breast Cancer

✌ Lymph node involvement at the time of breast cancer diagnosis is associated with increased risk of relapse. In the past, most women with lymph node involvement were offered chemotherapy. New studies indicate that women with Luminal A breast cancer with one to three involved lymph nodes still have an excellent survival rate with estrogen-directed therapy alone and get minimal benefit from chemo-therapy. To confirm the excellent prognosis despite limited lymph node involvement, genomic testing can be performed and has been validated in this 1–3 positive lymph node group of women with Luminal A cancers.

In summary, women with Luminal A breast cancer have an excellent prognosis with surgery or radiation and estrogen-directed therapy, even with lymph node involvement. Chemotherapy has essentially no role in this subtype of early breast cancer, and the utilization of hormone-directed therapy prior to surgery is becoming more prevalent. The choice and type of hormone-directed therapy should be tailored to each individual woman's situation. Both tamoxifen and aromatase inhibitors are effective choices but have different side effects.

Luminal B Breast Cancer

Luminal B breast cancers are hormone-positive but more aggressive than the Luminal A subtype. As presented in Table 8.1, these cancers are higher-grade and more proliferative, as shown by the elevated Ki67 after immunohistochemistry staining. In many cases, chemotherapy can be utilized before or after surgery to improve survival, which is then followed by hormone-directed therapy. Flow diagram 8.3 describes how we manage Luminal breast cancer at Breastlink. The treatment of Luminal B cancer requires a multidisciplinary approach with a pretreatment plan in place based on each patient's individual clinical situation.

The Role of Chemotherapy in Luminal B Breast Cancer

In the past, most women with Luminal B cancer were offered chemotherapy before surgery (neoadjuvant) or after surgery (adjuvant). However, not all women with Luminal B cancer benefit from chemotherapy, and with the development of genomic assays that predict risk of recurrence and benefit of chemotherapy, we are able to determine which women should be considered for chemotherapy

Test	Company	Number of Genes	Measure
Oncotype DX	Genomic Health	16 + 5 controls	RS low (<18), intermediate (18–31), high (>31)
MammaPrint	Agendia	70	Good risk and poor risk
Prosigna	Nanostring	50 + 22 controls	Low (<10), intermediate (10–20), high (>20)
Breast Cancer Index	Biotheranostics	5 + 2 gene ratio	Low, intermediate, and high risk of recurrence H/I ratio likelihood to respond to hormonal therapy

Table 8.2

Genomic assays for assessment for risk of recurrence

treatment. Table 8.2 lists a few of the current genomic tools available to oncologists for risk assessment and possible chemotherapy benefit.

With the advent of these important tools we have decreased the number of women with Luminal B breast cancer who are treated with chemotherapy by approximately 30 to 40 percent. If a genomic test indicates a woman's cancer is at significant risk of spreading into the bloodstream and might respond to chemotherapy, we then determine the most appropriate and beneficial schedule of chemotherapy for her—before surgery (preoperative/neoadjuvant) or postsurgery (adjuvant), as we discussed in chapter 6. The advantages of chemotherapy before surgery include

• Reducing the size of the primary tumor and allowing for less surgery and possible breast conservation

- Eradicating possible disease in the lymph nodes, potentially sparing more extensive lymph node surgery
- Gaining the ability to directly observe the effect of the drugs on the cancer
- Undertaking systemic treatment sooner, which is valuable when microscopic cells have escaped

In our experience, about 15 percent of Luminal B breast cancers identified by genomic testing, and their high-risk clinical features, completely disappear after surgery with no visible disease under the microscope. As previously mentioned, we call this a *pathologic complete response* (pCR), which translates into high chance of cure. If a women does not have a pCR after preoperative therapy, it does not mean she will not be cured. For most women with an incomplete response, we can study the cancer and decide on alternative chemotherapy after surgery or move on to hormonal therapy.

Chemotherapy Regimens for Luminal B Breast Cancer

✽ Over the last twenty-plus years, a number of clinical trials have tested various chemotherapy regimens in Luminal B breast cancer. Presently, most oncologists use one of several protocols (see chapter 6). We use a combination of docetaxel (Taxotere) with cyclophosphamide (cytoxan), known as TC, every three weeks, for four to six treatments. For high-risk women with positive lymph nodes, many oncologists will add doxorubicin (Adriamycin) to the TC. Unfortunately, doxorubicin includes risk of two rare but serious side effects: heart damage and leukemia. The risks and benefits of this chemotherapy regimen is an important conversation to have with your oncologist.

Hormonal Treatment for Luminal B Breast Cancer

Following local control and chemotherapy for high-risk women and local control for women whose genomic testing results indicate chemotherapy is not required, hormonal therapy is prescribed for a minimum of five years. As with Luminal A cancer, for premenopausal women, tamoxifen is the drug usually prescribed. For high-risk, young, premenopausal women with aggressive cancers who receive chemotherapy, an alternative approach is ovarian suppression combined with an aromatase inhibitor for five years. This approach is based on two recent clinical trials conducted in Europe that demonstrated a small but significant survival advantage over tamoxifen alone in the high-risk group. The criteria for this approach would be young women under age forty who require chemotherapy and have aggressive disease.

What Is the Best Hormonal Treatment for Luminal B Cancer?

A number of clinical trials have been conducted comparing tamoxifen and aromatase inhibitors in postmenopausal women with early Luminal breast cancer. It should be noted that these trials included both Luminal A and B patients. A meta-analysis, which is a combining of all significant randomized trials into one analysis—this one involving almost 32,000 women—shows a small survival advantage at ten years of about 2 percent favoring AIs over tamoxifen. There was no significant difference in outcome for women given tamoxifen for two to three years followed by an AI and for those receiving an AI for five years.

I suspect AIs have greater benefit in the Luminal B group than in the Luminal A group. In our centers we tend to recommend AIs for high-risk Luminal patients or to start with tamoxifen and switch after two years to an AI. I believe that women with high-risk Luminal B cancers are better able to tolerate the side effects of the AIs if they understand the risk/benefit. We aggressively try to address and mitigate potential side effects early on, especially joint aches, and we obtain a baseline bone-density study and monitor carefully for bone loss, treating with an anti-osteoporosis regimen when indicated.

Neoadjuvant Hormonal Treatment

✿ In the event that preoperative hormonal therapy is prescribed (usually when genomic testing indicates little potential benefit from chemotherapy), clinical trials support the use of an AI over tamoxifen in the postmenopausal patient. In premenopausal women there are few clinical trials reported in the literature, but the same principles that apply to postmenopausal women should also apply to younger women. Tamoxifen is given with or without ovarian suppression. Once ovarian suppression has been accomplished, tamoxifen may be replaced by an AI. The purpose of preoperative hormonal therapy is to shrink the cancer in the breast and lymph nodes and allow for a better surgical outcome. Studies show a 40 percent increase in breast conservation in women who would have required a mastectomy.

Length of Hormonal Treatment in Luminal B Breast Cancer

✿ I believe five years of adjuvant hormonal therapy is sufficient for the majority of women with Luminal A breast cancer. In Luminal B cancer, extended hormonal therapy may provide some survival advantage, as suggested by the European studies mentioned above. To determine if an individual will benefit from extended therapy, the BCI can also be used for Luminal B cancers to predict the risk of recurrence after five years of therapy and whether continued hormonal therapy will be effective. This test has also been very helpful in allowing women to feel confident stopping therapy after five years if they fall into the low-recurrence category.

In summary, Luminal B breast cancer requires a multidisciplinary approach and pretreatment planning based on staging, pathology, special IHC staining, and genomic testing. Some women will benefit from chemotherapy either before or after surgery, as determined by genomic analysis. *All* women with Luminal B breast cancer should receive a minimum of five years of hormonal therapy. AIs appear to be modestly better than tamoxifen in ten-year breast cancer survival but two to three years of tamoxifen followed by an AI appears to be equivalent. For lower-risk Luminal B patients, preoperative AI therapy can be utilized to reduce the size of the cancer for possible breast conservation and can be given to women with locally advanced cancer or women who are poor surgical candidates.

Clinical Research in Luminal Breast Cancer

✂ Research to determine why some Luminal breast cancer patients relapse and develop resistance to hormonal therapy has increased dramatically. With the ability to sequence the individual breast cancer genes, a number of mutated genes have been identified that cause resistance to hormonal therapy such as tamoxifen or aromatase inhibitors. Now that genes such as PTEN, PI3K, and CDK2,4/6 have been identified as carrying mutations that cause resistance, scientists have developed drugs that overcome the resistance and allow the hormonal therapy, in combination with these new agents, to be effective in eradicating the cancer.

Numerous clinical trials are testing the addition of new treatments in patients who are receiving traditional adjuvant hormone treatment. Some of the trials provide neoadjuvant hormonal treatment plus one of the new agents (see chapter 13) to women who have localized Luminal breast cancer. This yields almost immediate results showing the increased effectiveness when the new drugs are added. This is a very

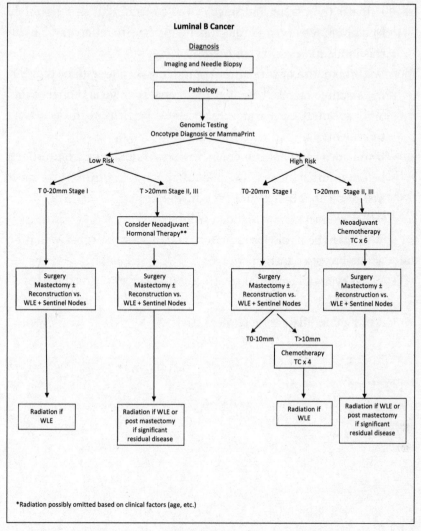

Flow diagram 8.3

Management of Luminal B breast cancer at Breastlink

exciting time in the treatment of this subtype of breast cancer, and I believe it will lead to major progress in its cure.

In conclusion, if you have been diagnosed with Luminal B breast cancer based on pathologic and genomic features of the biopsy, the following issues should be addressed for treatment planning:

- What is the extent and stage of the cancer? This is determined by a physical exam and imaging, including a mammogram, an ultrasound, and possibly an MRI.
- Will chemotherapy be necessary to increase cure rate by preventing systemic relapse based on your cancer's stage and phenotype?
- Will an analysis of your cancer genes be helpful in discussing treatment?
- If you are a candidate for chemotherapy, should it be administered before or after surgery? (Would an attempt to shrink the cancer first result in a better surgical outcome?)
- What chemotherapy regimen will be used?
- Will there be a role for radiation, and, if so, what type? Will it be whole breast or intraoperative?
- What type of hormonal treatment after surgery is recommended and for how long?
- Am I a candidate for a clinical trial?

Management of HER2-Positive Breast Cancer

Tremendous progress has been made in the treatment of HER2-positive breast cancer. This subset of breast cancer accounts for 15 percent of invasive breast cancer. If you are reading this chapter because you have been diagnosed with HER2-positive breast cancer, there is good news and bad news for you. The good news is that it is highly likely you will be cured. During the last fifteen years, the cure rate has gone from 50 percent and will soon exceed 90 percent. The bad news is that you most likely will require targeted anti-HER2 therapy with chemotherapy. In this chapter, we will briefly discuss local control and sequencing of treatment. We will also go over the science of this type of breast cancer and what distinguishes it from the other breast cancer types. The unique mutations causing this cancer have led to the development of targeted antibody therapies that have greatly improved survival. We will briefly explain these agents, their history, and how we use them. Progress has been so rapid in the treatment of HER2-positive breast cancer that before this edition is printed, there may be a new discovery or a new drug available for testing.

The reason your oncologist will probably prescribe systemic therapy for you is that HER2-positive cancers tend to be very aggressive and can spread into the bloodstream early, even when the cancer is small and

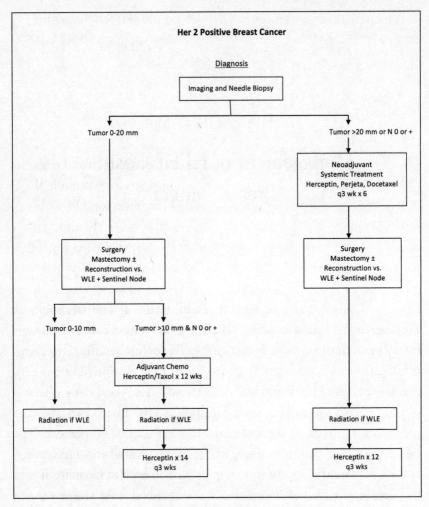

Flow diagram 9.1

Management of HER2 breast cancer

less than 20 millimeters. The systemic therapy, which is a combination of anti-HER2 agents and chemotherapy, is highly effective in eradicating any cells that have escaped and generally is well tolerated.

About one half of HER2-positive breast cancers can be also hormone receptor (HR) positive. Oncologists call these cancers "triple positive." If your cancer is triple-positive your oncologist will most likely prescribe hormone therapy after the completion of the anti-HER2 chemotherapy treatment. Figure 9.1 is a flow diagram of how we manage HER2-positive at Breastlink.

HER2 Positivity *Definition*

❦ This aggressive type of breast cancer, that we discussed some in chapter 3, is caused by a mutation on chromosome 17. Normally there is one HER gene on this chromosome and one receptor, but with the mutation multiple HER genes are formed that cause the production of multiple receptors on the cell surface. In fact, there are four HER receptors: Her1, HER2, Her3, Her4. These receptors trap a variety of growth factors circulating in the blood. Growth factors serve a number of functions in the body such as promoting wound healing, cell division, and so on. But once trapped by the cancer cell, the growth factor stimulates the cell's malignant processes further.

Development of an Anti-HER2 Drug

❦ Once scientists discovered the HER receptors and their active participation in the malignant process, Dr. Axel Ullrich at Genentech and Dr. Dennis Slamon developed an antibody to the HER2 receptor using a rat immune cell. Through an involved process, they were able to transplant the rat antibody DNA into a human immune cell and then produce large amounts of antibody in tissue (all cultured outside the body in a lab). They named the antibody trastuzumab, or Herceptin. Experiments demonstrated that Herceptin disrupted the malignant process and caused the cancer cell to self-destruct—what we call *apoptosis*. Herceptin was even more effective if it was added to chemotherapy. This was a monumental breakthrough, a "targeted treatment" that used antibodies that were directed and attached to the malignant cells.

Clinical Trials

⚥ As we will discuss in chapter 13, the process of bringing a newly discovered drug to the woman who needs it for survival is a painfully slow and rigorous process. Herceptin was FDA-approved in 1998 for women with stage 4 disease (cancer that had spread beyond the breast). It was found to be relatively safe but to have some effect on the heart, which could be monitored and was reversible. My patients and I have participated in these trials over the last twenty years, and I would like to thank all of the women who agreed to participate in the clinical trials. Because of you, the science has come so far today.

Herceptin added to chemotherapy after surgery was found to decrease systemic recurrence in 2006. Oncologists began giving the regimen before surgery (neoadjuvant), and about half of the women had no remaining disease in the surgical specimens removed from their breasts or lymph nodes—a pathologic complete response (pCR). This pCR highly predicts that the women are cured and there will be no relapse.

A second anti-HER antibody was developed that prevented the HER2 and Her3 from combining and forming a very potent, cancer-generating agent. The drug, pertuzumab (or Perjeta), was found to be synergistic with Herceptin and was approved for use for stage 4 cases in 2012. When Perjeta was given with Herceptin and chemotherapy in the neoadjuvant setting, the pCR rate increased by 20 percent. Perjeta was approved by the FDA for use before surgery in 2013.

Chemotherapy and Herceptin (and recently Perjeta) are given every three weeks for a total of six treatments, and then Herceptin alone is continued every three weeks to complete one year. Several trials were conducted to determine the optimal length of Herceptin treatments. In the Phare trial, six months of Herceptin was slightly inferior to twelve months, but there was significantly more cardiac toxicity in the women given Herceptin for a full year. At the American Society of Clinical Oncology (ASCO) meeting in June 2017, results of the Short-Her Study compared nine weeks of Herceptin with one year or fifty-two weeks of Herceptin combined with the chemotherapy. Participants (1,253 women) were randomized into one of two groups (nine weeks versus fifty-two weeks), and at five years there was no difference in overall survival. Researchers also found a 2.1 percent difference in *disease free* survival that favors the group treated with Herceptin for one year. Women with larger cancers and multiple involved lymph nodes benefited from the longer treatment period. As in the Phare trial, there were significantly more cardiac events in the longer treatment group (ninety cardiac events in the fifty-two-week group versus thirty-two in the nine-week group). The cost of Herceptin is significant: approximately $50,000 for fifty-two weeks, and $8,400 for nine weeks of treatment. I believe that the Phare and Short-Her studies show us that it is reasonable for women with early HER2-positive cancers (stage 1 and early stage 2 disease) to receive a shorter-duration Herceptin regimen. This is especially reasonable for older women with heart disease. One additional study, the Hera trial, compared one year versus two years of Herceptin and found that there was no benefit to extending Herceptin treatment beyond one year and that there was increased cardiac events in the group treated for two years.

In 2015, a lower weekly dose of Herceptin plus the chemotherapy drug paclitaxel (Taxol) was given to 410 women with early HER2-positive breast cancer after surgery for twelve weeks and then Herceptin for a year total. To qualify for the study, women had to have a cancer less than 3 centimeters and no involved lymph nodes. After three years, 98.7 percent of the patients were well without recurrence. These results were so phenomenal that the regimen called the APT, or the Dana-Faber regimen, has become widely prescribed.

Toxicity from the Herceptin regimens can cause cardiac effects that must be monitored but are almost always reversible once the Herceptin is complete. The chemotherapy that is combined with the Herceptin and Perjeta is usually a taxane, either docetaxel (Taxotere) or pacli-taxel. The taxanes cause bone marrow suppression, temporary hair loss, and reversible neuropathy. Doxorubicin (Adriamycin) is active, but because it has cardiac toxicity that is additive and more serious than that of Herceptin, it is used infrequently. Carboplatin, a drug that was used in the first postsurgery adjuvant trial with docetaxel and Herceptin (TCH), is being used less frequently. As you can see from flow diagram 9.1, we use the weekly Herceptin/Taxol for stage 1 can-cers after surgery; for stage 2 cancers (larger than 2 cm and/or with positive lymph nodes), we give neoadjuvant Herceptin, Perjeta, and docetaxel.

There are a number of other anti-HER2 drugs that are either approved in the metastatic setting or are in the clinical trial process. None of these will be offered to you outside a clinical trial. One of these agents, Kadcyla (ado-trastuzumab emtansine), is very interesting. It is Herceptin that is linked to a potent chemotherapy drug. The complex finds the cancer cell HER2 receptor via Herceptin, and then the potent chemo-therapy is deposited into the cancer cell with little or no exposure to normal cells. There are a number of clinical trials observing Kadcyla use in early breast cancer.

HER2 Testing

✁ Since the HER2-positive breast cancers require targeted, expensive drugs, it is critically important that accurate testing is done to deter-mine that indeed the breast cancer is HER2-positive. The standard testing involves an immunohistochemical (IHC) stain of the cancer cells' membranes. This is an antibody-fluorescent stain highly sensitive to the HER2 receptor. The staining intensity is graded by the patholo-gist. If there is little or no staining—a score of 0 or 1+—then the cancer is deemed HER2 negative. If the membranes are fully stained, they receive a score of 3+ and are deemed HER2 positive. The cancers that have intermediate stain (2+) require further testing using another technique, which looks at the ratio of HER2 mutations on chromosome 17 of the cell compared with other areas of the 17th chromosomes away from the HER2 location. This test is called a FISH (fluorescent in situ hybridization) test.

Most of the time this is sorted out accurately, but in about 5 percent of cases there is ambiguity. There may be areas within the tumor that have a different appearance (heterogeneity), or the ratios of HER2 counts to 17th chromosomes may vary. In these unclear cases we will request a second opinion from a breast pathologist who specializes in HER2 testing. There are false positives involving staining techniques. If a cancer under the microscope appears Luminal, low-grade, and is not behaving clinically like a HER2-positive cancer, we will repeat the IHC stain, redo the FISH test, or employ one of the newer versions of the FISH test that demonstrate increased amounts of the HER2 protein. These tests are very expensive at this time and are only used to sort out these rare ambiguous cases.

Sequencing of Treatment

✺ Since a majority of women with HER2 breast cancer will require HER2-antibody-based chemotherapy, the first question that comes up is whether it should be done before or after a local control method. In our clinics we do systemic therapy before local control if the cancer is bigger than two centimeters or if there is a positive lymph node. If the cancer is smaller than two centimeters, we will consider surgery, and the patient will often receive the weekly APT regimen postoperatively. One of the advantages of doing systemic therapy first is that if the patient does not have a pCR with the neoadjuvant regimen, then they may be eligible for postoperative trials involving newer anti-HER2 drugs.

Summary

✄ If you have HER2-positive breast cancer, your prognosis is excellent. Make sure the HER2 testing is correct and is congruent with the rest of your pathology. This area of breast cancer treatment is changing rapidly. In the last two years, Perjeta has been added to the treatment of early disease with excellent results. Kadcyla is also waiting in the wings, and there are a number of new agents in clinical trial testing. It is a very dynamic field, and you may want to seek a second opinion regarding your options.

10

······

❧

Management of Triple-Negative Breast Cancer

As we discussed in chapter 3, triple-negative breast cancers account for approximately 15 percent of all invasive breast cancers. These cancers are termed *triple-negative breast cancer* (TNBC) because their cell membranes lack receptors for estrogen, progesterone, and HER2.

The TNBCs are actually a diverse group. Based on gene expression, researchers have divided TNBC cancers into at least four subtypes. The majority fall into the *basal-type* (not to be confused with basal-type skin cancers), so you may see *triple-negative* and *basal-type* used interchangeably. We will discuss the nonbasal triple-negative breast cancer subtypes later in the chapter.

If you are reading this chapter because you have TNBC, be forewarned that the Internet is a scary place to go for information, and it's often old and inaccurate. There has been major progress in the last several years in our understanding and treatment of the TN subtype. It is true that TNBCs tend to occur in younger women; they are often fast-growing and are therefore discovered as a palpable breast mass rather than through breast screening.

Triple-negative breast cancer is associated with the BRCA1 gene. It is important for women who are diagnosed with TNBC to undergo genetic testing, since approximately 10 percent will have inherited the BRCA1 mutation. If you are BRCA1 positive, your risk of developing another breast cancer in the future is increased. Thus many women usually consider bilateral mastectomies to reduce the risk of future breast cancers. Another consideration is the increased risk of ovarian cancer, which is approximately 30 percent, so we recommend that women have their ovaries and fallopian tubes removed after child bearing.

For reasons still being studied, over half of breast cancers in African American women are TN, compared to 15 percent in Caucasian women. TNBCs also appear to be genomically different in African American women than in white women, with less BRCA1 positivity and lower responsiveness to traditional chemotherapies.

Unlike the Luminal and HER2 subtypes, the triple-negative breast cancers do not have specific targets on the cell surface at which to direct therapy, like hormone or HER2 receptors. This is changing, however, with the ability to explore genomic differences in the TNBC group. I predict we will have some specific targets, and targeted agents to employ in treatment, in the near future. As described above, a majority of triple-negative breast cancers are the basal subtype. They are quite proliferative, with high Ki67 scores and a high mitotic rate. This makes them very sensitive to chemotherapies that damage and kill rapidly dividing cells. Once damaged by chemotherapy, these cancer cells are often unable to make the DNA repairs needed to survive. Noncancerous cells in our bodies can easily repair themselves and return to health.

Neoadjuvant Chemotherapy

✻ Triple-negative cancer often presents as a rapidly enlarging breast mass, often larger than two centimeters in diameter at diagnosis. Since we can make the diagnosis with a needle biopsy and fairly accurately determine the stage by imaging and a physical exam, women today are often treated with chemotherapy before surgery to remove the cancer.

This is called *preoperative chemotherapy*, or, more commonly, *neoadjuvant chemotherapy*. The advantages of this approach are similar to those of any neoadjuvant treatment:

1. Therapy that treats the breast cancer locally and targets any cells that may have potentially escaped the breast can be started rapidly.
2. The cancer within the breast will reduce in size, making local control with surgery less deforming.
3. Lymph node involvement often decreases, allowing the surgeon to remove fewer lymph nodes, which reduces risk of arm swelling, or *lymphedema*.
4. There will be visible evidence that the chemotherapy is effective, as the cancer in the breast shrinks with treatment. A majority of triple-negative breast cancers will become undetectable by physical exam or imaging.
5. The possibility of complete disappearance of the cancer on microscopic examination of removed tissue at the time of surgery (pCR). This has a high correlation to cure.
6. The use of neoadjuvant chemotherapy has become an important research tool to test innovative regimens, using the pCR as the end point of the studies. In the past, we treated patients with chemotherapy *after* surgery, and research outcomes were not available until several years after the trials were completed, since successful outcomes were based on the absence of recurrence over time.

Because TNBC cells rapidly divide, cells that escape and are not destroyed by chemotherapy will usually present as metastatic lesions in the body within thirty-six months after treatment. This is different from the Luminal subtypes, which, if they recur, tend to do so much later than triple-negatives.

Flow diagram 10.1 describes how we manage triple-negative breast cancer at Breastlink centers.

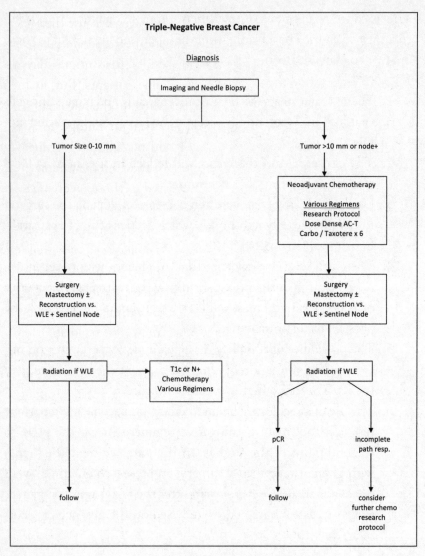

Flow diagram 10.1
Management of triple-negative breast cancer

The choice of chemotherapy regimens for triple-negative breast cancer varies depending on the institution and the treating oncologist. Many U.S. oncologists will follow guidelines set by the National Comprehensive Cancer Network (NCCN). There is often a time lag before the NCCN adopts new guidelines, however, because the NCCN breast cancer committee relies on completion of randomized clinical trials, which can take years to provide results. Institutions may also have research protocols in place for eligible patients. But, as mentioned above, neoadjuvant trials are speeding up the release of study results. An example is the GeparSixto trial in Europe in which Carboplatinum was added to the standard neoadjuvant regimen for TNBC. The women randomly assigned to the Carboplatinum group had a 20 percent increase in pCR compared to those receiving standard chemotherapy. Based on this result, it was evident that Carboplatinum is highly effective in killing TNBC by damaging the DNA of the actively dividing cancer cells. The damaged cells are unable to correct the DNA damage resulting in apoptosis, so this drug will very likely increase the cure rate. Many institutions are including Carboplatinum in their patient management, Breastlink among them, yet the NCCN guidelines do not currently contain this regimen.

The taxanes—docetaxel (Taxotere) and paclitaxel (Taxol)—directly interfere with the mechanism of chromosome migration as the cancer cell is dividing. The malfunction created by the taxane sends the cancer cell into apoptosis too. Carboplatinum combined with a taxane gives close to a 60 percent pCR when the regimen is administered prior to surgery.

Another drug, doxorubicin (Adriamycin), affects dividing cells and is frequently used in triple-negative breast cancer in both the adjuvant and neoadjuvant regimens, often coupled with cyclophosphamide (cytoxan), which damages the DNA. The two drugs are often administered every two weeks for four treatments along with a bone marrow growth factor (called dose-dense AC). This is often followed with a taxane regimen for twelve weeks. This sequence has been used for many years but is beginning to fall out of favor with the emergence of the Carboplatinum-taxane regimen. Less Adriamycin has been used in recent years because of several serious side effects, including damage to the heart and the rare increased risk of leukemia.

New Developments

As previously mentioned, a significant portion of young women who develop triple-negative breast cancer will have a BRCA1 mutation. This inherited mutation leads to a DNA repair defect in breast and ovarian cells. The repair defect prevents damaged breast and ovarian cells from recovering after treatment as they normally would, and this unrepaired damage can lead to the development of cancer. Women with BRCA1 mutation have approximately 60 percent lifetime risk of breast cancer and a 30 percent risk of ovarian cancer.

The defect that causes cancer in BRCA1 patients leads to a cancer that is particularly fragile and is unable to repair itself when exposed to chemotherapy. A group of newly developed drugs called PARP inhibitors also inhibit DNA repair, and when given with a chemotherapy drug like Carboplatinum, seem to increase the cell-killing effect by further preventing DNA repair. These PARP inhibitors are currently being tested in clinical trials, and two drugs have just received FDA approval to treat ovarian cancer in BRCA-positive patients.

Another group of drugs called *immune checkpoint inhibitors* (or PDL-1 inhibitors) are actively being tested in triple-negative breast cancers. This class of drugs has been responsible for the recent breakthroughs in melanoma and lung cancer treatment. These drugs neutralize a protein sent by the cancer to the immune system that inhibits the immune system from mounting an active response to the cancer. Currently at Breastlink, we are participating in a clinical trial using a checkpoint inhibitor in triple-negative breast cancer.

The Other Triple-Negative Breast Cancer Subtypes

As I previously mentioned, TNBCs are a diverse group and, although the basal subtype is by far the most common and the most chemotherapy-sensitive, there are other types, which are distinguished based on gene profiling. Chemotherapy is the treatment of choice for all subtypes, but targeted agents are being tested to better tailor treatment for these genomically different subtypes.

The four subtypes are

1. Basal-like 1 (BL1), the most common, is very chemosensitive and has a high pCR rate.
2. Basal-like 2 (BL2) is much less chemosensitive and is not associated with BRCA1 positivity.
3. Luminal androgen receptor type (LAR) is not really a triple-negative breast cancer and has an androgen receptor on its surface. It is chemosensitive with a pCR of 30 percent. Trials are looking at targeting the androgen receptor with drugs that are similar to those used in the treatment of prostate cancer. It has been observed that the LAR subtype has a large percentage of PI3K mutations, so there may be a role for recently developed PI3K-inhibitor drugs.
4. Mesenchymal stem-like (MSL) is the rarest subtype and has decreased proliferative genes and lower chemosensitivity compared to the others. Cells under the microscope can appear similar to sarcoma, or squamous cell cancers, which are referred to as "metaplastic." Recently these cancers have been found to make a unique protein (RPL39), which may lead researchers to develop new treatments.

If you are diagnosed with TNBC, do not panic. There is now real progress being achieved in the treatment of TNBC. Researchers are investigating genomic differences between the subtypes, which will ultimately lead to development of more targeted agents and better outcomes. Presently, chemotherapy is the primary treatment, often given prior to surgery and often resulting in a pathologic complete response. A number of new agents are being tested in clinical trials, especially in the neoadjuvant setting. If you have a TNBC you may want to investigate the possibility of a clinical trial (see chapter 13). I believe that in the near future, genomic testing will be routinely used in triple-negative breast cancer to aid in treatment planning and the selection of chemotherapy regimens.

II

. . . . . .

Risk Assessment and Genetic Testing

All cancer is genetic. That is to say, in order for a normal cell to change into a cancer cell, a genetic mistake must occur. These incidental or environmentally induced mutations are called *somatic mutations*. Another type of mutation can be inherited from a mother or father. These mutations pass from the egg or sperm and are called germ line mutations.

A majority of breast cancers are the result of somatic mutations, probably about 85 percent. The remaining 15 percent are the result of germ line mutations that an individual is born with and that predispose the person to develop cancer. These mutations often occur in genes responsible for the repair of somatic mutations. The repair genes act like watchdogs to keep us safe from developing cancer and may affect only certain organs or types of cells. For example, the BRCA1 mutation described below affects breast and ovary cells in women and prostate cells in men. The BRCA2 mutation is also associated with breast and ovarian cancer and, rarely, pancreas and stomach cancer.

Until recently, only these two germ line genes had been identified. BRCA1 (1st BReast CAncer gene) was discovered in the early 1990s, followed by the second breast cancer gene, or BRCA2. We knew there must be other genes with germ line mutations because of multiple families with major breast cancer prevalence that tested negative for BRCA1 and 2. Based on these family studies, we know BRCA1 and 2 account for about 40–50 percent of inherited breast cancer susceptibility. Since the last edition of this manual, there are now another fifteen genes identified that account for most of the other approximately 50 percent.

The other new development since the last edition of this manual is in the availability of genetic testing. One company, Myriad Genetics, previously retained exclusive rights to do breast cancer gene testing based in part on their claim that they controlled a patent in the breast cancer gene itself. However a new legal ruling has established that the gene itself could not be patented. Breast cancer gene testing is now done by multiple laboratories, and the cost has become much more reasonable despite the addition of almost twenty different breast cancer susceptibility genes. As a result, insurance companies have broadened the eligibility guidelines, allowing more patients to be tested.

It is important to understand that every person is born with two copies of every gene, one inherited from the mother and the other from the father. When a condition (in this case breast cancer) requires only one copy of a gene in order to have a mutation, it is called an *autosomal dominant trait*. If an individual inherits a germ line mutation from one of their parents, only half of their eggs or sperm (germ cells) will contain the mutation. Therefore, the children of a mutation carrier each have a 50 percent risk of inheriting the mutation and being affected. Both men and women can carry breast cancer mutations, so in charting family pedigrees it is important to study both sides of the family. We suggest gene testing is appropriate in the following situations:

1. Early-onset breast cancer (at under 45 years of age), regardless of family history of breast cancer
2. Male breast cancer at any age
3. Breast cancer and ovarian cancer in the same woman

4. Three or more breast cancer cases on the *same side* of the family, maternal or paternal side
5. Three or more breast, ovarian, or pancreas cancer cases on the *same side* of the family, maternal or paternal side
6. Bilateral breast cancer
7. Triple-negative breast cancer at under 65 years of age

We strongly recommend that when considering breast cancer gene testing you consult a genetic counselor. You can get a referral at most cancer centers, hospitals, and institutions that conduct the testing. Your physician can assist you in finding a genetic counselor who will help explain the implications of the test results and how it will affect your future choices.

The benefits of gene testing are multiple. A negative test means that you don't carry one of the approximately twenty currently known genes and your breast cancer is unlikely to be the hereditary type. A negative test also means that your children will not inherit a known breast cancer gene from you.

The criteria for referral to genetic testing as described above can help with decision-making as follows:

✓ If you have a positive gene test with a newly diagnosed cancer, you may want to base your surgery choices on your increased risk of a second breast cancer (e.g., prophylactic mastectomy).
✓ If you have a positive gene test without cancer, you may want to modify your surveillance options and possibly take risk-reduction measures, such as prophylactic oophorectomy (after childbearing) for women with inherited risk of ovarian/breast cancer.
✓ With a TP53 mutation, you should avoid radiation exposure.
✓ Testing allows you to inform other family members at risk of carrying the gene, too, so that they can make appropriate health care decisions.
✓ A positive gene test will help provide guidance and eligibility for new gene-specific therapies as they emerge.

A genetic counselor can be very helpful explaining the risks of a positive test and the possible interventions. Testing is accomplished quite simply with a blood test or cheek swab. Detailed information regarding the seventeen known germ line genes that cause 20–80 percent of one's lifetime risk of breast cancer is beyond the scope of this manual but can be obtained through genetic counselors, online resources, and the public domain. Known genes with greater than 20 percent lifetime risk are listed in Table 11.1.

A few more points on this topic are worth emphasizing. If you have a newly diagnosed breast cancer, I think it is important to create a family pedigree if possible. Germ line mutation carriers usually develop a breast cancer at an earlier age than women without a mutation, so young age is a red flag, as is bilateral breast cancer or the combination of ovarian and breast cancers on the same side of the family. There are great references for creating your own family health pedigree listed in the Resources section at the end of the book.

Remember that males and females inherit breast and ovarian cancer germ line mutations equally, but females usually manifest the cancer. Affected families that are predominantly men on the paternal side can go unrecognized as mutation carriers. A paternal aunt or grandmother can provide important clues in such cases.

Many women who discover a hereditary breast cancer gene either through a breast cancer diagnosis or through a family health pedigree

ATM	NBN	PALB2
BRCA1	RAD 50D, RAD51C, RAD51D	PTEN
BRCA2	CHEK2	P53
BARD1	CDH1	NF1
BRIP1	MUTYH	MREIIA

Table 11.1

Known genes with breast cancer risk greater than 20 percent

choose to have their breast tissue removed with bilateral mastectomies. The benefit of this choice is that risk of a new breast cancer diagnosis drops to nearly zero percent and the need for frequent surveillance (mammograms, MRIs, etc.) throughout their lives becomes unnecessary. If you are considering prophylactic mastectomies with reconstruction, be sure to find a team (breast surgeon and plastic surgeon) that do this procedure frequently and ask to see their work. The cosmetic results have become very good as surgeons have perfected their techniques and the prosthetic materials have improved. Nipples can now be preserved with little risk of harboring breast tissue, but unfortunately nipple sensation is lost.

The timing of prophylactic mastectomies is an important issue. If a woman with newly diagnosed breast cancer is found to be gene-positive, she often chooses mastectomy at that time. The advantage in this case is avoiding radiation, which makes future reconstruction less optimal. The cancer surgery and prophylactic surgery can be done simultaneously with matching reconstruction for symmetry and appearance.

Young women who are gene-positive but don't have breast cancer are in a different situation. I recommend annual surveillance with an ultrasound and a physical exam beginning at age twenty-five. I prefer not to do mammograms because the breast tissue at this young age is susceptible to radiation damage, and women with BRCA1 or BRCA2 lack a repair gene, as previously discussed. After age thirty, breast cancer risk begins to rise and many young women will choose surgery even without a cancer diagnosis. It is interesting that the risk of dying from breast cancer is about the same—very low—whether you have preventative surgery or move to a more vigilant surveillance program after age thirty, usually consisting of biannual checkups alternating mammograms with ultrasounds and MRIs. So the real choice here is whether a woman is willing to commit to frequent screening.

For BRCA 1 and 2 positive patients, the risk of ovarian cancer is 20–40 percent (the higher end of that range for BRCA1). Our surveillance for ovarian cancers is not as good as for breast cancers, so we usually recommend removal of the ovaries after childbearing. There is a risk of other, less common cancers associated with these genes (pancreatic cancer or melanoma, for example), and surveillance should be discussed with the genetic counselor.

12

Nutrition and Lifestyle

I know that many of you are anxious to read this chapter because you want to find out what you may have done to cause your breast cancer, what you can do to cure this cancer, or how you can prevent another breast cancer in the future. I speak with patients every day who tell me they think they caused their breast cancer through "bad" dietary choices. They believe they must make radical changes to prevent another breast cancer or cancer recurrence. I understand these feelings; this is a time when many people feel out of control, and wanting reasons for what happened and straightforward solutions is completely natural, and having them would be very comforting.

The reality is that there is no nutrient or group of nutrients that caused your breast cancer. And unfortunately no nutrients can prevent or cure cancer; there is no magic bullet. It is very important to understand you did not cause your breast cancer and you cannot cure it by changing how you eat or how you live. That said, you *can* use this event as a defining moment in your life to make changes that will help reduce your future risk of cancer and reduce your risk for other health conditions, all of which will help you lead a long, healthy, and active life.

Quite popular now online, on television, and in numerous publications are testimonials suggesting that breast cancer can be prevented and even cured through diet and lifestyle changes. There are hundreds of so-called "experts" who pass along misleading and unscientific information about breast cancer cures. Many have products for sale and try to make money off a vulnerable population. Unfortunately, some of these approaches do have an understandable appeal, since they are often simple to comprehend and put into practice, which is empowering.

Create Your Lifestyle Plan

✻ In this chapter I will present nutrition and lifestyle recommendations that are based on the best scientific knowledge available today, designed to help you contribute to your overall treatment plan. This is where you have absolute control over how you will live a healthy lifestyle! Earlier chapters described the importance of creating your personal treatment plan and finding the best treatment team of radiologists, surgeons, oncologists, and other specialists. But until now, we have not discussed the most important member of your treatment team: YOU! Every member of your team has evaluated your unique situation and developed a plan for how they will address your care. We are now at the point where we call on *you* to evaluate your own health and lifestyle and begin developing a plan that identifies the choices you will make to live a healthy and active life as a breast cancer survivor.

Nutrition and lifestyle play an essential role in your breast cancer journey. Eating a wide variety of foods daily will help you to stay healthy, retain energy and strength, enhance your immune system, promote growth of healthy cells, and *contribute* to reducing risk of cancer or cancer recurrence. Being physically active will help you to achieve and maintain a healthy body weight, improve mood, boost energy, and promote better sleep. Engaging in regular physical activity will also help to prevent or manage a wide range of other health conditions such as diabetes, cardiovascular or heart disease, high blood pressure, stroke, metabolic syndrome, and it will help to maintain strong bones, too!

Prehabilitation

I am particularly excited by research in the area of cancer *prehabilitation*, which is defined as "a process on the cancer continuum of care that occurs between the time of cancer diagnosis and the beginning of acute treatment." Until recently, in the United States it has been rare for oncologists to begin hormonal or other chemotherapy treatment prior to surgery, but as we've seen, this is changing. It has now become much more common for patients to receive preoperative treatment for three to six months or, rarely, up to a full year. This period of time between diagnosis and beginning treatment is the ideal opportunity to develop and implement healthy lifestyle changes. You have time now to evaluate your current lifestyle and make healthy changes that are not cures but that can reduce your risk for the rest of your life.

A prehabilitation program can help you to

- Learn about cancer-risk-reduction strategies
- Make lifestyle changes to improve your health and fitness
- Develop and implement a healthy lifestyle plan and set achievable goals for the future

The importance of incorporating physical fitness into your prehabilitation plan cannot be emphasized enough. A growing body of evidence shows that breast cancer patients who improve their physical fitness levels *before* beginning therapy are better able to tolerate treatment and recover faster. Research also suggests not only that exercise is safe *during* cancer treatment but also that it can improve physical functioning and self-esteem and reduce fatigue and anxiety. It also helps heart and blood vessel fitness, muscle strength, and body composition (the ratio of fat to bone to muscle mass).

Breast Cancer Risk Factors

As previously noted, the purpose of a healthy lifestyle plan is to *reduce risk* and to improve quality of life before, during, and after cancer treatment. Let's begin by examining the factors that *increase risk* of breast cancer. The strongest risk factor for breast cancer is age; risk for developing breast cancer increases as we get older, and we can't change this. However, research shows that there are additional factors that increase risk, some of which are within our control.

Factors that increase risk of breast cancer that we *cannot* change:

- Being female
- Reproductive and menstrual history
- Family history of breast cancer
- Genetics (for example, having BRCA1, BRCA2, or other gene mutations, though these account for no more than about 10 percent of all breast cancers)
- Race (in the United States, breast cancer is diagnosed more often in white women than in African American, Hispanic, Asian, or Native American women)
- Long-term use of menopausal hormone therapy (combined use of estrogen plus progestin for more than five years)
- Dense breast tissue
- Personal history of breast cancer

Factors that increase breast cancer risk that we *can* change:

- Being overweight or obese
- Maintaining a low level of physical activity
- Consuming too much alcohol
- Smoking

Addressing the factors that you can change to reduce your risk of breast cancer should be the focus of your lifestyle plan. Of course, creating and implementing a lifestyle plan may be difficult when you are in the midst of your cancer diagnosis, but this is an opportunity for real change. You are in control! And that can take you out of patient mode and put you into active participant mode. How will you go forward in your life now to make a difference in your care and recovery?

Take a quick survey of your current lifestyle:

Are you maintaining a healthy body weight?
Do you follow a regular physical activity program?
Are you consuming more alcohol than you should?
Do you smoke?

Achieve and Maintain a Healthy Body Weight

Compelling evidence indicates that being overweight or obese (having a body mass index [BMI] over 25) increases risk of breast cancer, especially after menopause. Being overweight can also increase risk of breast cancer recurrence and more than ten other cancer types. Type 2 diabetes, metabolic syndrome, heart disease, high cholesterol, and hypertension are all associated with being overweight or obese. If you are reading this manual and you have been diagnosed with breast cancer, *lifestyle choices* are where you have the most control over your health.

What is a healthy body weight? We use BMI most often as a quick calculation that measures a person's body fat. Because the calculation is based on body weight and not on body composition, BMI does not take into account how much of a person's weight is from muscle, bone, water, or fat. This means, for example, that a person with more muscle mass and strong bones (say, an athlete) may have a high BMI but not be overweight or obese. At the same time, an older adult who has lost muscle mass might have a deceptively low BMI. It is just one way to assess weight that may or may not indicate overall wellness, and of course it does not tell us anything about a person's fitness level.

In spite of this, we use BMI most often because it is a quick screening tool that most medical practitioners agree is useful. The guidelines for determining whether someone is overweight or obese are not hard-and-fast, and combining BMI with another assessment, such as waist circumference, often provides a more accurate risk appraisal for obesity-related disease. Men with waist circumferences of greater than forty inches and women with circumferences of more than thirty-five inches are at greater risk for developing conditions such as insulin resistance, metabolic syndrome, heart disease, and other conditions.

To calculate BMI:

weight (pounds) divided by height (in inches) squared, multiplied by 703

You can also go to an online BMI calculator for adults, plug in your height and weight, and your BMI will be calculated instantly. See those provided by the National Institutes of Health (www.nhlbi.nih.gov /health/educational/lose_wt/BMI/bmicalc.htm) and Centers for Disease Control and Prevention (www.cdc.gov/healthyweight/assessing/index .html). Or ask your health clinic, physician, or other medical staff to calculate your BMI while you are in the medical office.

What weight category are you in?

Weight Category	BMI
Underweight	Less than 18.5
Normal	18.5 to 24.9
Overweight	25.0 to 29.9
Obesity	30.0 to 39.9
Extreme Obesity	40.0 or higher

Table 12.1
BMI weight categories
based on adults age 20 and older

The first thing I tell most newly diagnosed breast cancer patients is not to gain weight. Now, if your BMI is below 18.5, you are most likely underweight and this recommendation would not apply, and you should see your physician or a registered dietitian nutritionist for a complete assessment. For everyone else with a normal BMI or higher, one of the important things you can do to stay healthy is to make a plan to avoid gaining weight.

Relationship Between Body Fat and Breast Cancer

✂ Research suggests several different ways in which being overweight or obese might affect cancer risk:

- People who are overweight or obese often have low-level, long-term, or *chronic*, inflammation, and over time this may cause DNA damage that leads to cancer and cancer recurrence. Researchers who study the link between inflammation and breast cancer risk believe that obesity-linked health conditions such as type 2 diabetes or heart disease can also lead to long-term inflammation, which may further increase risk of breast cancer recurrence or even death. For this reason many researchers are interested in whether anti-inflammatory medications, such as aspirin or nonsteroidal anti-inflammatory drugs, reduce the risk of cancer.
- In addition to obesity, chronic inflammation may also be caused by infections that don't go away or abnormal immune reactions to normal tissues. For this reason many researchers are interested in whether anti-inflammatory medications, such as aspirin or nonsteroidal anti-inflammatory drugs, reduce the risk of cancer. However, research to date has yet to establish a clear answer to this intriguing question.
- Fat tissue produces excess amounts of estrogen, high levels of which have been associated with increased risk of breast and other cancers.

- Overweight and obese people often have increased levels of insulin and insulin-like growth factor-1 (IGF-1). This condition, known commonly as insulin resistance, occurs before a diagnosis of type 2 diabetes. High levels of IGF-1 may promote certain cancer types.
- Fat cells produce adipokines, hormones that may stimulate or inhibit cell growth. For example, leptin is an adipokine that seems to promote cell growth, and as the amount of body fat increases, the amount of leptin in the blood also increases, which encourages the growth of cancer cells.
- Excess fat tissue can also cause changes in breast tissue cells, immune responses, and oxidative stress (imbalance between the production of free radicals and the body's ability to neutralize their toxic effects through production of antioxidants), all of which affect risk for cancer.

Breast Cancer and Weight Gain

Stress can cause many folks to reach for the nearest high-calorie comfort foods, and, as we can all agree, breast cancer diagnosis is stressful. Also, as we age, it is not unusual to gradually start adding pounds, so be aware of this and develop strategies to minimize weight gain. Additionally, women who have been diagnosed with breast cancer often report subsequent weight gain. Some in the medical field believe it is due to different cancer medications and treatments, the onset of menopause, or changes in body composition. Current research is mixed on the mechanism that results in weight gain in breast cancer patients, and while some patients do gain weight, others do not, which further complicates the issue. Interestingly, weight gain is seldom seen with other types of cancer; in these cases we typically find that weight loss is the biggest concern.

For those of you in the normal BMI weight group, make a plan to maintain your weight through treatment and beyond. It is much easier to stay at your current body weight than to try to lose added pounds later on. Having a plan in place *prior* to beginning treatment will help improve your chances of maintaining a healthy body weight. Being mindful of the food choices you make combined with regular physical activity will contribute to keeping your weight in a healthy range.

If your BMI category is overweight or above at diagnosis, plan to maintain your weight, but also begin exploring different lifestyle choices and strategies that you can use to help you reach your ultimate healthy lifestyle goals.

I don't think I'm telling you anything new when I say that losing weight is very difficult and keeping it off can be even harder, particularly since genes play a role in determining body type and how much you will likely weigh throughout your lifetime. However, since our goal is to reduce your risk of breast cancer and cancer recurrence, there are recommendations about how to achieve and maintain a healthy body weight with that specific goal in mind:

- Health professionals often suggest aiming for 5 to 10 percent weight loss. While this target weight may leave you in the "overweight" or "obese" range, it can still very effectively decrease your risk for chronic diseases related to obesity. (For example, if you weigh two hundred pounds, losing 5 to 10 percent of your body weight would be a 10 to 20 pound weight loss; your goal weight would be 180 to 190 pounds.)
- After reaching your goal weight, try to maintain it. This period of maintenance is highly variable and unique to the individual; it may last for only one month or for much longer. Once you feel absolutely confident that you can maintain your new weight, you can move forward to set a new goal and work to get there.
- Develop a plan for being physically active every day, in any way, and stick to it! Your physical fitness level can improve no matter what you weigh, and it will have dramatic health benefits. Besides reducing risk for cancer and many other health conditions,

physical activity can help reduce fatigue, strengthen the immune system, and, of course, burn calories.

If nothing else, try your best not to gain weight. It will complicate your treatment, be very difficult to lose later, and will increase your risk of cancer recurrence as well as risk of other health conditions.

How Did We Get Here?

As in all other aspects of your breast cancer care, we must rely on science to show us the way. We know from the tremendous advances in breast cancer treatment over the past forty years that science is constantly evolving and improving. This includes nutrition science, as well.

In the 1960s the general focus was on the role that food carcinogens might play in increasing cancer risk. Carcinogens are chemicals produced at high temperatures; such as when meats are grilled or barbequed, that are known to produce DNA mutations in animal models. There may be some truth to this theory; however, if carcinogens do play a major role in cancer risk, we have had more than forty years for more solid evidence to surface.

In the 1980s and 1990s, the focus was on *dietary fat* (the fat we consume in our diet) as the major cause of cancer. For people with conditions such as diabetes and heart disease, monitoring dietary fat intake is very important. However, research data does not support the idea that increased calories from dietary fat will increase cancer risk.

When it became apparent that dietary fat was not responsible for increasing cancer risk, the focus shifted to fruits and vegetables for risk reduction. Unfortunately, the idea that consuming more fruits and vegetables would dramatically reduce cancer risk has not been supported by subsequent scientific research either. This is not to say that consuming fruits and vegetables is unimportant, and in fact there probably is some cancer-risk-reduction benefit from consuming plant foods, but it is likely a small benefit.

The evidence today is overwhelming: excess body fat is a major cause of cancer. We refer to excess body fat as *positive energy balance* because people who consume more calories than they burn through physical activity will store the excess calories as body fat (adipose tissue), which translates into weight gain. Compare this with *negative energy balance*, where fewer calories are consumed than are burned, which results in weight loss. This is actually a pretty straightforward process; no matter how complicated it can seem, weight loss and weight gain come down to calories in versus calories out.

The evidence that excess body fat contributes to cancer comes from an overwhelming number of research studies conducted over the past ten to fifteen years. It's interesting to note that as early as the 1930s, animal studies suggested that excess body fat contributed to cancer; it just took us a while to return to this concept!

The Healthiest Way to Eat

We are bombarded with the enormous number of diets and meal plans available online and in magazines, and it seems like new strategies burst onto the scene every day. Promoters of these plans scream from the rooftops that they've found the diet solution to cure what ails you! One plan will encourage complete elimination of certain nutrients while another touts the importance of consuming only raw foods. There's the low carbohydrate diet and the high protein diet, the cabbage soup diet or blood-type-specific diet. Some preach that you should eat like a caveman, count every calorie, or never count calories at all. So how do we sort out what's true and what will actually help you stay healthy?

Virtually all of these plans have one thing in common: they are all low in calories. So if you follow them exactly, you will likely lose weight, if that is your goal. The important questions are, Will you be able to keep the weight off? Is the diet compatible with your lifestyle? Is this really the *healthiest* way to eat? Research shows that it's pretty unlikely any of these diet plans will have a permanent place in your life because, frankly, they are unsustainable. They are complicated and often unpleasant, and they do not promote a healthier way of eating that will benefit you long term.

Plus, adhering to complex meal plans can be stressful, and stress is not good for you. The constant examination and evaluation of every meal that you eat is exhausting and does not even ensure that you are consuming all of the nutrients you need to reduce your risk of chronic disease. So I am giving you permission to relax. Eating a healthy diet is not so tricky. You don't need to count calories (unless you want to), you don't need to shop at specialty stores or buy expensive kitchen appliances, and you don't need to feel guilty that you're not following the latest fad.

Before we discuss specific recommendations for healthy eating, let me first say that no matter the meal plan you choose, you must take it and make it your own. If you don't customize it in a way that works for you, it will not work. It will become too difficult or boring, and you will most likely stop. No matter how you choose to go about this, the very best meal plan is one you can stick to.

With this in mind, eating healthfully is not complicated—that is, unless you want it to be! Some people are happiest when the level of complexity is high—when there is a lot to think about and talk about and investigate. They like to feel like they are "going the extra mile." These folks may want to follow a meal plan that is very detailed and explicit and may even be the latest diet craze.

At the other end of the spectrum are people who hope that eating a healthy diet won't be too different from their current habits. Maybe they don't have the time or energy to put out additional effort toward making different food choices or changing their status quo. They prefer easy-to-follow suggestions and little fuss. That said, the majority of us fall somewhere in between these two extremes.

Be sure to recruit team members who will participate and support you in your healthy lifestyle. If you have a busy and active household, this can be the core of your team. Friends and coworkers are also very important. Research shows that people with the strongest support from others have an easier time making changes. By modeling healthy behavior for loved ones and friends, you will impact their lifestyles as well, even if they don't appear to "buy in" right from the beginning. Change is a slow process. If you just keep doing what you are committed to, I guarantee it will become a part of you and have an impact on those around you.

MyPlate, New American Plate, and DASH Diet

Of the hundreds of different meal plans available, I have chosen three that I believe are excellent guides to eating healthfully and that are easy and straightforward to follow. These programs are anchored in the philosophy that to reduce risk of chronic disease, Americans should begin by eating a wide variety of foods from the five food groups every day while increasing the amount of plant foods in the diet (fruits, vegetables, and whole grains). This does not mean consuming only plants; instead, the recommendation is to fill your plate one-half to two-thirds full with plant foods while including fewer foods containing saturated fats, sugar, and salt.

The first plan, MyPlate was developed by the United States Department of Agriculture (USDA) as a tool to help you find *your* healthy eating style and build on it throughout your lifetime. Everything you eat and drink matters. This means:

- Focus on variety, amount, and nutrition.
- Choose foods and beverages with less saturated fat, sodium, and added sugars.
- Start with small changes to build healthier eating styles.
- Support healthy eating for everyone.

Healthy eating is a journey shaped by many factors, including stage of life, preferences, access to food, culture, traditions, and daily routines.

MyPlate offers ideas and tips to help you create a healthier eating style that meets your individual needs, improves your health, and, most important, reduces your risk of disease. Go to www.choosemyplate.gov to get started.

In partnership with MyPlate, the USDA has developed Super-Tracker, a tracking tool that can help you plan, analyze, and track your diet and physical activity. Find out what to eat and how much; track your intake, physical activity, and weight; and personalize with goal setting, virtual coaching, and journaling. These great tools are available on the USDA website at no cost for anyone who wants to reduce risk of chronic disease and live a healthier lifestyle. Years' worth of research consistently shows that people who track what they eat and how much they exercise have an easier time sticking to their program and achieving their goals (www.choosemyplate.gov/tools-supertracker).

A second option, the New American Plate, was developed by the American Institute of Cancer Research (AICR) and is very similar to the USDA MyPlate program. According to the AICR, the New American Plate is not a diet or a complex system for calculating calories, fat grams, or carbohydrates. It's a fresh way of looking at what you eat every day. You can create meals that lower your risk for cancer and other chronic diseases and manage your weight at the same time. As described on the AICR website, the New American Plate should be made up of two-thirds (or more) vegetables, fruits, whole grains, or beans (plant foods) and one-third (or less) animal protein.

Essential to all healthy eating plans is the idea of *portion control*. Over the years American waistlines have grown larger and larger, keeping pace with the ever-increasing portion sizes we manage to consume. For this epidemic there is a simple solution: eat smaller portions! If you want to decrease your weight and reduce risk of disease, develop strategies to consume less food. For example, serve meals on smaller plates, don't have junk food or sugary beverages in the house, and eat a full serving of vegetables *before* every meal to fill you up and reduce hunger so you won't need seconds!

What is an appropriate serving size? There are many online resources available that describe serving sizes for just about any food you can imagine. The following table describes standard serving sizes for the different food groups and provides a visual aid for what the serving size looks like.

Standard Serving Sizes

And finally, one of my favorites, the Dietary Approaches to Stop Hypertension (DASH) meal plan. The DASH diet is similar to both

Food	Serving	Looks Like
Chopped Vegetables	½ cup	½ baseball
Raw Leafy Vegetables (such as lettuce)	1 cup	1 baseball or adult fist
Fresh Fruit	1 medium piece ½ cup chopped	1 baseball ½ baseball
Dried Fruit	¼ cup	1 golf ball
Pasta, Rice, Cooked Cereal	½ cup	½ baseball
Ready-to-Eat Cereal	1 oz., varies from ¼ cup to 1¼ cups	
Red Meat, Poultry, Seafood	3 oz. (boneless cooked weight from 4 oz. raw)	Deck of cards
Dried Beans	½ cup cooked	½ baseball
Nuts	⅓ cup	Level handful for average adult
Cheese	1½ oz.	4 dice or 2 9-volt batteries

Table 12.2

Standard serving sizes

MyPlate and the New American Plate in that the primary focus is once again on plant foods. While the original idea developed over twenty years ago was a research study to help decrease hypertension, DASH has since gone mainstream, having been named numerous times as the best overall eating plan in annual nationwide surveys of health care providers. Lots of information can be found on the Internet about DASH and at the website for the National Heart, Lung, and Blood Institute (NHLBI), which helped develop the program. Once you have calculated your daily calorie needs, DASH shows you how many servings per food group you should eat every day (www.nhlbi.nih.gov/health/health-topics/topics/dash).

Physical Activity and Exercise

✀ Dozens of recent research studies have shown that women who are physically active have a 30 to 40 percent lower risk of breast cancer than their sedentary peers. Estrogen seems to play a key role in this distinction: women with high estrogen levels in their blood have increased risk for breast cancer, and since exercise lowers blood estrogen, it helps lower a woman's breast cancer risk, too.

Physical activity may prevent tumor development by

- Reducing hormone levels
- Reducing other cancer-growth factors such as insulin and insulin-like growth factor-1 (IGF-1)
- Improving the immune response
- Helping achieve and maintain a healthy body weight
- Helping lower BMI and excess body fat

Women of all ages should be concerned about becoming active and staying active. Physical activity has been associated with a reduced risk of breast cancer in both premenopausal and postmenopausal women; however, the evidence is somewhat stronger for postmenopausal breast cancer. Studies show that increased physical activity can decrease the risk of breast cancer by approximately 20 to 40 percent. In addition, physical activity has been associated with increased life expectancy in the general population as well as in women who have been diagnosed with breast cancer.

According to national activity guidelines, a good goal is to exercise at least thirty minutes a day most days, if not every day, of the week. Ideally, you should aim to accumulate at least 150 minutes of moderate endurance activity every week. While it sounds like a lot, 150 minutes is only two hours and thirty minutes per week, or about the same amount of time you might spend watching a movie. The good news is that you don't have to do it all at once. You can break it up over the day as long as you do moderate or vigorous intensity for at least ten minutes at a time. Moderate-intensity activities such as brisk walking are sufficient, although more benefit can be gained with increased intensity.

There is convincing evidence that even moderate activity can be critically important in helping reduce the risk of cancer, heart disease, and other chronic ailments. Physical activity reduces fat deep in the abdomen ("intra-abdominal" fat), a hidden risk factor because it can raise insulin levels, which promotes the growth of cancer cells. Most American women gain one to two pounds on average every year, and that adds up to dangerous levels over a lifetime.

In addition to reducing the risk of cancer, researchers have established that regular physical activity can improve overall health by

- Maintaining healthy bones, muscles, and joints
- Reducing risk of high blood pressure, heart disease, diabetes, and premature death
- Promoting psychological well-being

Despite these amazing health benefits, recent studies show that over 50 percent of Americans do not engage in enough regular physical activity.

The beauty of exercise as a method to reduce total and intra-abdominal fat—and therefore chronic disease—is that it can be done by most everyone at low cost and with low risk of side effects. It's never too late to enjoy the health benefits of exercise!

Here are a few tips to help get you moving:

1. **Reduce screen time.**
   - Screen time means television screens, computer monitors, and even the handheld devices we use for checking email, listening to music, watching TV, and playing video games.
   - Health experts say screen time at home should be limited to two hours or less a day! The time we spend in front of the screen, unless it's related to work or homework, could be better spent being more physically active (increasing energy burned).

2. **Make time to be active.**
   - Identify the best free time for you during the week.
   - Select the physical activity you like best and add it to your daily routine. For example, walk or ride a bike, walk the dog, exercise while watching TV, park a little further from your office, store, or library to get in a nice walk.
   - Take a walk during your lunch hour or take fitness breaks instead of coffee breaks. Try doing something active with your family or friends after dinner or on weekends.
   - Check out activities requiring little time. Try walking, jogging, or climbing stairs for ten minutes in the morning, afternoon, and evening for a total of thirty minutes every day.

3. **Stay motivated.**
   - Plan ahead. Make physical activity a regular part of your schedule. Write it on your calendar.
   - Join an exercise group or class.
   - Pick activities requiring no new skills, such as walking or climbing stairs.
   - Exercise with friends who are at the same skill level as you.
   - Wear a pedometer every day and track your steps. Once you

have begun increasing your steps, gradually increase until you reach ten thousand steps (five miles) per day.

- Start where you are. Set achievable goals and increase slowly until you arrive at your highest personal goal.
- Walk to visit coworkers or friends instead of calling or sending email.
- When the weather doesn't cooperate, grab a friend and take a walk in the local mall.

Changing Behavior

Making changes is hard. Not everyone is ready or in the right place to make lifestyle changes right now, and that's okay. You are reading this chapter for some reason, so at the very least you are thinking about it, which is great!

I think of this challenging time as an opportunity for you, a time when you can take charge of your health and your future. Of course, your first goal is most likely to never face a cancer diagnosis again, but lifestyle changes made now can also help prevent additional health-related conditions that may be waiting down the road such as heart disease, diabetes, or hypertension.

Because change is almost universally difficult to achieve, health care practitioners often describe it as a process with a series of stages. What stage are you in?

Stage 1: Precontemplation

During this stage, you may recognize that you should adopt a healthier lifestyle or that you would like to lose weight, but perhaps you ignore the problem and tell yourself that it's not a big deal. In this stage, you may not recognize that you need to make changes or you're not interested.

Stage 2: Contemplation

❧ In this stage, you become more aware of your habits and spend time thinking about your situation. Although you are able to contemplate change, you tend to be ambivalent about it. At this point, you're weighing the pros and cons of making a change but are not committing to it. This stage may take as little as a week or as long as a lifetime!

Stage 3: Preparation/Determination

❧ Now, you've committed to making change and you're motivated. You begin taking small steps toward change, such as cleaning junk food out of your cupboard, recruiting an exercise buddy who will hold you accountable to your shared routine, or exploring new websites for healthy, low-fat meals. If you skip this stage and jump from Contemplation to Action, you will probably struggle to stay committed. Making major lifestyle changes is hard. Take your time!

Stage 4: Action/Willpower

❧ At this stage you actively take steps to live a healthier lifestyle. You follow healthy habits at mealtime by watching portion sizes and eating more plant foods, and you're reducing stress by finding an exercise routine that you really enjoy and can stick with. You are also getting friends and family involved in this journey, and you are learning to enjoy yourself and have fun. If there isn't some fun, you risk boredom, which is one big reason why people fail to stay on track.

Stage 5: Maintenance

❧ During this final stage, your focus is on the new healthy behaviors you have adopted that have gotten you where you are. You developed a plan of action to achieve your goals. Understand that you will have bad days, but it is so important not to punish yourself. Don't give up— get right back out there! By adopting this new lifestyle, you have become healthier and stronger right from the beginning. Be sure to reward your successes—just not with food!

Vitamin, Mineral, and Herbal Supplements

❧ We need a variety of nutrients each day to stay healthy, including calcium and vitamin D to protect our bones, folic acid to produce and maintain new cells, and vitamin A to preserve a healthy immune system and vision. While getting our nutrients from a pill sounds like an easy solution, supplements don't necessarily deliver on the promise of better health.

At this time there is no scientific evidence that vitamin, mineral, or herbal supplements can prevent cancer. The few clinical trials testing whether supplements can reduce cancer risk in humans have all had disappointing results, and a few trials have found that high-dose supplements may actually increase cancer risk. A diet rich in vegetables, fruits, and other plant foods may have some effect on reducing cancer, but there is no proof that dietary supplements can reduce cancer risk.

There are some situations where supplements are recommended:

- Vitamin D and calcium for good bone health
- Vitamin B-12 in older people who may no longer absorb it
- Folic acid in women of childbearing age
- Individuals who have been told by their doctor that they have a specific nutrient deficiency

Vitamin A

Vitamin A is needed to maintain healthy body tissues. It is obtained from food in two ways: from animal food sources or plant sources. In the case of the latter, our bodies can make vitamin A from beta-carotene (or other carotenoids) obtained from foods such as sweet potato; carrots; dark-green, leafy vegetables; squash; cantaloupe; sweet red pepper; dried apricots; and peas or broccoli. Vitamin A supplements have not been shown to lower cancer risk, and high-dose supplements may, in fact, increase the risk for lung cancer in current and former smokers.

Vitamin C

Vitamin C is found in many vegetables and fruits, especially oranges, grapefruits, and peppers. Many studies have linked intake of foods rich in vitamin C to a lower risk of cancer. But the few studies in which vitamin C has been given as a supplement have not shown to reduce risk of cancer.

Vitamin D

Growing evidence suggests that vitamin D may help prevent colorectal cancer but so far does not support links to other cancers. Large studies about vitamin D and other cancer types are now under way, but the results will not be ready for several years. The Institute of Medicine recently increased recommendations for the daily intake of vitamin D, based on levels required for bone health, from 400 to 600 international units (IU) for most adults and to 800 IU per day for those seventy years and older. The upper daily limit of what is considered safe was increased from 2000 IU to 4000 IU.

Vitamin D is obtained through skin exposure to ultraviolet (UV) radiation, through diet, especially products fortified with vitamin D such as milk and cereals, and from supplements. But many Americans do not get enough vitamin D and are at risk of deficiency, especially people with dark skin or who get little sun exposure, as well as the elderly and exclusively breastfed babies (since bottle formula is usually fortified with vitamin D).

Vitamin E

Alpha-tocopherol is the most active form of vitamin E in humans and a powerful antioxidant. In one study, male smokers who took alpha-tocopherol had a lower risk of prostate cancer compared with those who took a placebo. This led to a large study (known as SELECT) that looked at the effects of selenium and vitamin E supplements on prostate cancer risk. But the study found that these supplements did not lower the risk of prostate cancer. If anything, the men taking vitamin E supplements may have had an increased risk.

Another large study (known as HOPE) looked at the risk of cancer and heart disease in people taking vitamin E supplements versus a placebo. No difference was seen in cancer rates or heart disease rates between the groups. Heart failure rates were actually higher among those taking vitamin E supplements.

Therefore, vitamin E supplements are *not* recommended to lower risk of cancer or chronic diseases, although foods containing vitamin E, including nuts and some unsaturated oils, can be healthy and have been shown to lower the risk of heart disease.

Soy Foods

⚘ Soy and foods derived from soy are an excellent source of protein and a good alternative to meat. The current consensus among health experts who study soy is that breast cancer survivors can safely eat these foods. Emerging research suggests that soy foods may *decrease* the likelihood of breast cancer recurrence in women with a history of the disease, although the evidence is not yet strong enough to recommend that all women with a history of breast cancer eat more soy. Soy foods do appear to be safe and possibly beneficial for female breast cancer survivors. Whether this applies to foods that contain soy protein isolates (protein powder, bars, or shakes) or textured vegetable protein derived from soy (soy meat, soy chunks, soy flour) is not known. However, there is little data to support the use of supplements of isolated soy phytochemicals to reduce cancer risk.

Tea

✺ Tea is a drink that results from infusion of the leaves, buds, or twigs of the tea plant (*Camellia sinensis*). Black, green, white, and other varieties of tea all come from the same plant but reflect the different ways in which they are processed. It has been proposed that tea might protect against cancer because of its antioxidant, polyphenol, and flavonoid content. In animal studies, some teas (including green tea) have been shown to reduce cancer risk, but findings from studies in humans are mixed. The results of some lab studies have been promising, but evidence at this time does not support drinking tea to reduce cancer risk.

Water

✺ The amount of water you consume every day plays an important role in maintaining a healthy body. Experts recommend drinking eight to ten glasses of water each day to maintain good health. Water helps keep your body hydrated, which is essential because almost every cell in the body needs water to function properly. If you dislike plain water, try sugar-free, fruit-flavored water or add a slice of lemon.

Other fluids such as milk, juice, and tea also count toward your daily total. Foods high in water such as lettuce (95 percent), watermelon (92 percent), and broccoli (91 percent) can help replenish lost fluids. It is important to drink plenty of water while undergoing chemotherapy, in particular.

Turmeric

❧ Some research is under way to examine whether turmeric can affect cancer growth. Other spices also being studied for possible anticancer effects include capsaicin (red pepper), cumin, and curry. At this time, there are no human studies that look at the long-term effects of spices on cancer and other diseases.

Sugar

❧ Sugar increases calorie intake and provides no nutrients that reduce cancer risk. Eating a high sugar diet actually promotes obesity. White (refined) sugar and unrefined sugar or honey are the same with regard to their effects on body weight or insulin levels. Limiting foods such as cakes, candy, cookies, and sweetened cereals, as well as sugar-sweetened drinks such as soda and sports drinks, can help reduce calorie intake and weight gain.

Artificial Sweeteners

❧ At this time, there is no scientific support for the idea that artificial sweeteners, at the levels consumed in human diets, cause cancer, despite various claims found on the Internet and reported in popular media. Aspartame, saccharin, and sucralose are a few of the artificial sweeteners approved for use by the FDA. Current evidence does not show a link between these compounds and increased cancer risk. Some animal studies have suggested that their use may be linked with an increased risk of cancers of the bladder and brain or of leukemias and lymphomas, but studies in humans show no increased cancer risk. People with the genetic disorder phenylketonuria, however, should avoid aspartame in their diets.

Newer sugar substitutes include sweeteners such as sugar alcohols (sorbitol, xylitol, and mannitol) and naturally derived sweeteners (stevia and agave syrup). All of these sweeteners appear to be safe when used in moderation, although larger amounts of sugar alcohols may cause bloating and stomach discomfort in some people.

Organic

The term "organic" is widely used to describe foods from plants grown without adding artificial chemicals and from animals raised without hormones or antibiotics. Organic plant foods come from farming methods that do not use most conventional pest or weed killers, chemical or sewage-sludge fertilizers, or food irradiation in processing. Foods that are genetically modified cannot be called organic.

While the purpose of organic food production is to promote sustainable farming practices, it is widely perceived that eating organic foods may carry health benefits. There is some debate over whether organic produce may have higher nutritional levels than conventionally grown produce, but at this time there is no evidence that such foods are more effective in reducing cancer risk or providing other health benefits than similar foods produced using other farming methods.

Processed Meat

Some studies have linked eating large amounts of processed meat to increased risk of colorectal and stomach cancers. This link may be due in part to nitrites, which are added to many lunch meats, hams, and hot dogs to maintain color and to prevent bacterial growth. Eating processed meat and meat preserved using smoke or salt increases exposure to potential cancer-causing agents and should be reduced as much as possible.

Irradiated Foods

✄ There is no proof that irradiation of foods causes cancer or has harmful human health effects. Radiation is increasingly used to kill harmful germs on foods to extend their shelf life. Radiation does not stay in the foods after treatment, and eating irradiated foods does not appear to increase cancer risk.

Garlic

✄ Claims of the health benefits of the *Allium* compounds found in garlic and other vegetables in the onion family have been publicized widely. Garlic is now being studied to see if it can reduce cancer risk, and a few studies suggest that it may reduce the risk of colorectal cancer. Garlic and other foods in the onion family may be included in the variety of vegetables that are recommended for lowering cancer risk. At this time, however, there is no evidence that *Allium* compound supplements can lower cancer risk.

Coffee

✄ Recent studies examining a possible link between coffee and cancer of the pancreas have not been confirmed. At this time, there is no evidence that coffee or caffeine increases the risk of cancer.

Antioxidants

✄ The body uses antioxidants, which are compounds found in foods, as well as in chemicals made in the body, to help protect against tissue damage that happens constantly as a result of normal metabolism (oxidation). Because such damage is linked with increased cancer risk, some antioxidants may help protect against cancer.

Antioxidants include vitamin C, vitamin E, carotenoids (such as beta-carotene and vitamin A), and many other phytochemicals (chemicals from plants). Studies suggest that people who eat more vegetables and fruits, which are rich sources of antioxidants, may have a lower risk for some types of cancer. But this does not necessarily mean that it is the antioxidants that are responsible for this, since these foods also contain many other compounds.

Several studies of antioxidant supplements have not found that they lower cancer risk. In fact, some studies have found an increased risk of cancer among those taking supplements. (See also entries for beta-carotene, and vitamin E supplements.) To reduce cancer risk, the best advice at this time is to get your antioxidants through food sources rather than supplements.

Alcohol

Alcohol raises the risk of cancers of the mouth, throat, voice box, esophagus, liver, breast, colon, and rectum. People who drink alcohol should limit their intake to no more than two drinks per day for men and one drink per day for women. A drink is defined as twelve ounces of beer, five ounces of wine, or one and a half ounces of 80-proof distilled spirits (hard liquor). The combination of alcohol and tobacco increases the risk of some cancers far more than the effect of either drinking or smoking alone. Regular intake of even a few drinks per week is linked to a higher risk of breast cancer in women.

Smoking

Don't smoke.

13

Clinical Research Trials

Progress in treatment and cure of breast cancer has been painfully slow. Fortunately, due to accelerated research programs and development of new treatment options, we appear to be entering a new era in cancer diagnosis and treatment. Funding from private philanthropies, the U.S. government, and private industry sponsors has driven all areas of breast cancer research, and the results are very promising. Understanding that breast cancer is due to a number of genetic mutations, scientists have refocused their efforts on finding ways to target therapy that can reverse or eliminate malignant cells within the body. This type of therapy is very different from the toxic chemotherapies that were the mainstay of adjuvant therapy in the past.

In the last several years, we have seen the new targeted therapies trastuzumab (Herceptin) and pertuzamab (Perjeta) become the standard treatment for *HER2-overexpressing* breast cancer. Lapatinib (Tykerb) is moving quickly through the testing process and will soon be used in early *HER2-positive cancers*, as well as Kadcyla, which is the first linked-antibody chemotherapy drug for breast cancer. Everolimus (Afinitor) and palbociclib (Ibrance) are targeted agents against DNA mutations and are being tested in early Luminal breast cancer.

In triple-negative breast cancer, a number of PDL-1 inhibitors are also in the clinical trial process.

All of these drugs, as well as many more in the research pipeline, are specifically targeted at the mutated cancer cell, leaving the normal, healthy cells alone. Besides drug development, clinical research involves the development of new therapeutic and diagnostic procedures. These new technologies are expensive and must be proved to be safe, helpful, and cost-effective. Sentinel lymph node sampling, MRI, PET scanning, and genomic risk assays are a few examples of technologies that are now part of standard breast cancer care.

Treatment changes can only occur after physicians and their patients are convinced that a new treatment or procedure is superior to what is already available. This process of demonstrating whether a new therapy is better than the previous standard therapy requires that women volunteer to participate in the testing of new medications and treatment options. Such projects are known as *clinical research trials.* Research trials must be conducted in an unbiased, fair way so that the results are reliable and the rights of the patient are protected. This requires that women be randomly entered into different treatment groups. Eventually, the outcomes of each group in the trial are compared against one another. For example, data drawn from past clinical trials have provided the following important results:

- Less surgery plus radiation is as effective as mastectomy in stage 1 or 2 breast cancer.
- Giving chemotherapy to women with local breast cancer prevents the development of metastatic disease.
- Tamoxifen and aromatase inhibitors given after surgery increase the cure rate in women with hormone-positive breast cancer.
- A negative sentinel lymph node predicts the rest of the axillary lymph nodes will be negative.

The randomized clinical trial eliminates physician and investigator bias, an important issue in trials comparing new therapy with standard therapies. The major breast cancer research group in the past has been the NSABP (National Surgical Adjuvant Breast and Bowel Project). This group includes surgeons and radiation and medical oncologists from all parts of North America and has combined with the national radiation oncology and gynecologic oncology groups to form NRG Oncology. Before the merger, the NSABP had conducted more than thirty-five randomized trials in breast cancer over the past thirty-five years. In recent years there has been a movement to increase scientific cooperation among breast cancer researchers around the world. Clinical trials are now coordinated internationally so there is less repetition of similar trials and the research is more timely and cost-effective.

Patients who have been willing to participate in clinical research studies have made a significant contribution to medical progress for all of society. Each trial tests a new hypothesis, or theory, and the results then become the knowledge base for the next clinical trial. In order to show significant differences in therapy, several thousand women are needed as volunteers in each trial. The volunteers realize that they may be getting the established treatment or the experimental treatment, and they will most likely not be told which they are receiving. They bravely participate with this degree of uncertainty. These pioneer women agreed to go into clinical trials comparing mastectomy to lumpectomy or a new chemotherapy regimen to the established one. These women didn't know if one treatment was more or less effective than the other, but they agreed to help answer the research question, Which therapy is optimal?

Today, research trials compare the standard of practice, or current state of the art, in breast cancer treatment, to what might *potentially* be better. The difference in treatment plans involves the sequencing of different therapies or the addition of a new drug. There are many opportunities to participate in clinical research trials in which you would receive state-of-the-art care. The National Cancer Institute (NCI) sponsors researchers around the United States and world including the NRG, Southwest Oncology Group (SWOG), and the Cancer and Leukemia Group B (CALGB). In order to participate in a clinical study, you must be willing to be randomly assigned to a treatment group. You will be asked to carefully read and sign a detailed informed consent document that explains the research purpose and procedures and the risks and benefits involved with participation. Many community-based oncologists participate in cooperative trials sponsored by the National Cancer Institute (NCI). If you are interested, you should discuss this option with your physician and treatment team. Information about clinical trials is available from NCI's Cancer Information Service at 1-800-4-CANCER and in the NCI booklet *Taking Part in Cancer Treatment Research Studies*, which can be found at http://www .cancer.gov/publications. This booklet describes how research studies are carried out and explains possible risks and benefits. Further information about clinical trials is available on the NCI website: http:// www.cancer.gov/clinicaltrials. The website offers detailed information about specific ongoing studies by linking to PDQ, NCI's comprehensive cancer information database.

In addition to clinical research trials, there are a number of small research projects available called *pilot studies*. These small studies are often designed to explore novel and cutting-edge ideas or therapies and are usually not randomized. They are often underwritten by pharmaceutical companies or entrepreneurial companies, and many are conducted at teaching hospitals and universities. As in all research, safeguards are in place to protect participating individuals to the greatest extent possible. Pilot study protocols are usually designed for women with advanced disease who are willing to place themselves at some increased risk because of limited available alternatives.

Human clinical trials are separated into four phases, depending on the questions that each one is attempting to answer:

- **Phase 1** testing is designed to determine if a promising treatment has acceptable tolerance in patients and at what dosage significant side effects appear. This phase usually involves a small group of participants (20–80). Once an agent, drug, or treatment has been proved safe, phase 2 testing begins.

- **Phase 2** involves a larger group (100–300) and further evaluates safety and quantifies the objective response rate (measures the reduction in cancer) resulting from use of the agent, drug, or treatment being tested. In women with breast cancer, both phase 1 and phase 2 testing are performed in patients with metastatic disease.

- **Phase 3** testing involves yet a larger group (1,000–3,000) and confirms the agent's or drug's effectiveness and how it compares with standard treatment. Information is collected that will allow the drug or treatment to be used safely. Most of the trials for women with newly diagnosed breast cancer are phase 3 trials. The clinical trial process of testing new therapy requires an orderly process that ensures safety and accuracy.

- **Phase 4** studies are done after the drug or treatment has been marketed to collect information on side effects associated with long-term use.

For many of us, physicians and patients, this process seems too slow. To speed things up, the world's breast cancer research community must collaborate and coordinate to eliminate duplication of clinical trial research. As more women enter trials, progress toward results will continue to increase.

We are very interested in testing promising new therapies in the *neoadjuvant* (preoperative) setting using the primary cancer's response as a marker of effectiveness of a new drug or treatment. If the primary cancer disappears completely, we know there is a high probability of cure. Research of this type allows for much faster progress because we do not have to wait years for a cancer recurrence to determine differences between treatment groups.

Another type of research trial is the large, *epidemiologic* (population-based) research study. These types of studies are not clinical trials.

Instead, they examine the cause, distribution, and control of disease (in our case, breast cancer) in populations. Groups, or populations, of people are examined to identify who is affected by a particular disorder; changes in incidence and mortality over time are studied; and associated risk factors are proposed. Epidemiologic data are used to recognize those groups at high risk for a disease and to recommend preventive measures that impact public health policies and future clinical trials research.

This type of research often relies on lengthy surveys about health and family history questionnaires, and sometimes on the collection of biospecimen samples such as blood or saliva or tumor tissue. Because epidemiologic studies are not clinical trials, they do not provide medical care or treatment, and you will probably not receive personalized results from any testing done using the information or samples you provide. Some of the things that breast cancer epidemiologists seek to identify include: (1) women within a population who may be at risk for developing breast cancer, (2) the geographic location where breast cancer risk is highest, (3) when the cancer will likely occur and trends over time, (4) exposures that breast cancer patients have in common, (5) how much the risk is increased through exposure, and (6) how many breast cancer cases could be prevented through elimination of the exposure.

Our advice is to ask your doctors if you are eligible for any research trials. Also inquire as to whether your providers participate as investigators in any studies or if there is a research center participating with one of the cooperative groups near you. Your ability to participate may depend on the type of health care delivery system you are in, so you will want to talk to your insurance company or HMO representative as well. In general, the next several years should prove very exciting in the field of breast cancer clinical research because enormous financial and scientific resources are being devoted to understanding the genetic mutations that lead to breast cancer and there is a large emphasis on the development of new agents aimed at prevention and cure.

14
. . . . . .
🌿

Life After Breast Cancer Diagnosis
BECOMING A SURVIVOR

If you are just beginning your journey with breast cancer, you may want to put this chapter aside for a while and come back once you get through your *acute treatment phase*—and you will! For most women, breast cancer is a life-altering experience. Statistically, you are joining three million U.S. women who are also survivors and with whom you share many experiences relating to this disease. This chapter addresses issues of survivorship: fear of recurrence and health screening; health maintenance such as bone health; hormonal concerns and sexuality; financial and insurance issues; spirituality and stewardship.

Fear of Recurrence and Health Monitoring

🌿 A majority of women are cured of their breast cancer—more than 80 percent! To me, *cured* means that you live the rest of your life without recurrence, and you die of something other than breast cancer, in the distant future and beyond your eightieth year. But we do not know with *absolute confidence* if you are cured. My hope is that by using this manual and with the help of your medical team you have received optimal treatment and you have given yourself the best possible chance. All survivors have some anxiety about recurrence. Early on, the everyday aches and maladies of living can rekindle this anxiety.

Risk of recurrence does decrease over time; however, there is no absolute amount of time that guarantees cure. One certainly celebrates five- and ten-year anniversaries. We know that women with triple-negative and HER2 types of breast cancer are usually safe after three years and that women with Luminal A or Luminal B cancers can relapse after five years but rarely after ten. I should point out that women who do relapse with metastatic disease often have long-term survival with current and evolving treatment strategies. The management and prognosis of metastatic breast cancer can be very similar to other chronic diseases of aging, such as diabetes, chronic lung disease, and heart disease.

A major controversy among the medical establishment is how closely survivors should be monitored for systemic recurrence. There is no question that survivors need annual breast screening to monitor for local recurrence or a second breast cancer. Women receiving adjuvant hormonal treatment such as tamoxifen or aromatase inhibitors are usually followed by their oncologist every three to six months with examinations and blood tests until the treatment is complete.

We do not believe in routine radiologic scanning (CT, PET, and bone scans) unless there is a persistent symptom or an abnormal blood test. We think that women with a history of breast cancer who have remaining breast tissue have a modest increased risk of a second breast cancer and require annual diagnostic mammograms. For women with increased breast density, MRIs are more effective than mammograms, but are expensive and the gadolinium dye used in the study may accumulate in the body. An alternative to MRI is whole breast ultrasound, which we recommend be added to an annual screening mammogram in women with dense breast tissue.

Bone Health

Bone health is a major issue for breast cancer survivors. It is important to be proactive in helping women protect their bone mass and guard against osteoporosis in later life. Breast cancer survivors have treatment issues that make them vulnerable to accelerated bone loss, including (1) chemotherapy and chemotherapy-induced menopause, (2) estrogen deficiency and the lack of hormone replacement therapy, (3) aromatase inhibitor (AI) treatment, and (4) vitamin D deficiency, which has been associated with breast cancer. It is important to monitor bone health in order to intervene appropriately. We recommend that our patients have a baseline serum vitamin D level and a bone density exam. We also advise taking supplemental vitamin D and calcium supplementation with lifestyle modifications, including smoking cessation and weight-bearing exercise.

Several drugs are beneficial for the treatment of osteoporosis, including the bisphosphanates (Fosamax, Boniva, Zometa) and a drug recently approved by the FDA, Denosumab. These drugs do have side effects. The bisphosphanates contribute to *gastroesophageal reflux disease (GERD)* and can rarely cause unusual fractures in the middle of the *femur* (thigh bone). Both classes of drugs can also lead to *osteonecrosis* of the jaw *(ONJ)*, although this too is rare. ONJ, when it occurs, usually follows a dental procedure such as a tooth extraction or root canal.

With *osteopenia* (significant bone density decrease but with no risk of fracture), we recommend conservative management with vitamin D and calcium supplementation and exercise. However, if a woman is on an AI, or if she continues to lose bone mass on the conservative treatment, we will add a bisphosphanate or Denosumab after a thorough baseline dental exam.

Gynecologic Health, Sexuality, and Hormone Replacement Therapy (HRT)

✤ There are often major concerns for the breast cancer patient around gynecologic issues, particularly for younger *premenopausal* or *perimenopausal* patients with Luminal A or Luminal B (hormone-receptor-positive) cancer who are receiving adjuvant hormonal therapy. It is estimated that as high as 50 percent of these patients will discontinue hormonal therapy (increasing their risk of recurrence) because of side effects, many of which are related to estrogen deficiency and menopausal symptoms.

The medical community should help women suffering from these unpleasant side effects before they *throw in the towel* on this very important and potentially lifesaving treatment. The AIs were first marketed by the pharmaceutical industry as superior to tamoxifen, and while the two classes of hormonal therapy are fairly equal in effectiveness, their side effects are different. Although it is true that the AIs don't increase the risk of *uterine hyperplasia* (a rare but serious side effect that can lead to uterine cancer) or increase the risk of *venous thrombosis* (a blood clot in a vein)—both of which are attributed to tamoxifen—the complete estrogen blockade caused by the AIs can lead to side effects that are intolerable for some women.

Common complaints are *arthralgias* (joint and muscle aches), loss of sexual desire, vaginal thinning, and vasomotor symptoms (hot flashes). For some postmenopausal women, tamoxifen in combination with vaginal estrogen can be a much better tolerated regimen in spite of the rare serious side effects that we can monitor for.

HRT in breast cancer survivors is a controversial and complex subject. In 2001 the Women's Health Initiative Study reported an increased risk of breast cancer in women taking a combination of estrogen and progesterone. The same study reported that women who'd had a hysterectomy and were taking estrogen alone had no increase in breast cancer, had increased bone density, had decreased incidence of colon cancer, and received no benefit in cardiovascular or Alzheimer prevention. Follow-up reports in 2009 further confirmed these findings.

The use of HRT in breast cancer survivors has been discouraged, especially in women who survived hormone-receptor-positive cancer. This is in spite of the fact that a vast majority (more than 80 percent) of these patients are cured. Added to this is my belief that if a woman has a systemic relapse after initiating HRT, the HRT has not caused the relapse. The cancer was there and may have recurred somewhat earlier because of the estrogen stimulation. What we need is a SERM-like hormone replacement that is safe to use in breasts and good for bone health. There has been some progress toward this goal: a combination medication of conjugated estrogen (Premarin) with a SERM drug (bazedoxifene) was recently released. This combination drug, brand-named Duavee, decreases breast density and increases bone density but does not stimulate the lining of the uterus. It improves menopausal symptoms. Whether it is safe for survivors of Luminal breast cancer has not been studied in a clinical trial.

In the meantime, the medical community should provide individualized, supportive therapy around quality-of-life issues for women who are undergoing adjuvant hormonal therapy or who are beyond active treatment. For some women, homeopathic remedies, herbs, and SSRIs are effective in controlling symptoms. For women who are so symptomatic that they are willing to abandon adjuvant tamoxifen or AI therapy in spite of the survival benefit, I will sometimes add low-dose estrogen to tamoxifen with excellent relief of symptoms (adding estrogen to AI therapy would counter its effect).

There is no clinical trial to support this approach, but I think it is worthy of closer evaluation. Theoretically, it should be safe (excluding uterine stimulation) because we know tamoxifen is effective in preventing systemic relapse in premenopausal women who are producing their own estrogen.

Fertility

❧ For young women with breast cancer, fertility can be a very important issue! As modern women delay childbearing, breast cancer can suddenly jeopardize a woman's or a couple's ability to have children. A large percentage of young women have hormone-negative cancer (triple-negative or HER2-positive) requiring chemotherapy but not requiring long-term hormonal therapy that would cause an extended delay of pregnancy. Chemotherapy can affect endocrine function (hormone production) of the ovary in premenopausal women receiving this therapy. The degree of the dysfunction depends on the intensity and type of chemotherapy and the health and age of the woman's ovaries.

In my experience, most women under age thirty-five will have transient interruption of ovulation due to the chemotherapy exposure. Usually within six months and rarely up to one year after completing chemotherapy, ovulation and menstrual cycling resume. Women entering their forties have fewer remaining eggs and older ovaries, and their fertility may be more affected by chemotherapy: there is a small but real chance of permanent cessation of ovulation and menstrual periods (premature menopause). Egg harvesting with embryo storage is an option.

Our policy is to offer premenopausal women interested in fertility the opportunity to see a gynecologist who specializes in fertility medicine. If patients elect to undergo this treatment, there often will be some delay in beginning the breast cancer treatment, so it is important for physicians to make this referral as early as possible.

Stress and Breast Cancer

❧ Many of my patients ask me this question: "Dr. Link, did stress cause or contribute to my breast cancer?" And the follow-up question: "If the answer is yes, where does that leave me, now that I am even more stressed because of the cancer diagnosis!" In spite of considerable literature from the 1980s linking stressful events to a diagnosis of cancer, I do not believe that stress in any way causes breast cancer.

The old literature does not stand up to scientific scrutiny. While some animal studies have found a relationship between chronic stress exposure and decreased immune function, I do not believe that decreased immunity has a major role in the development of breast cancer. We do not know why women get breast cancer or why the incidence has increased substantially over the last thirty years, except in two instances. We know from epidemiologists that long-term exposure (greater than five years) to an estrogen/progesterone hormone replacement therapy combination increases a woman's risk of Luminal B breast cancer by about 20 percent.

We also know that women who have inherited one of the genes discussed in chapter 11 will have up to a 50 percent risk of developing breast cancer. But that's it. We do not know the causes for the remaining 80-plus percent of breast cancers. Life is stressful. Getting breast cancer is stressful. I believe continuous unrelieved stress is bad, and people who feel hopeless are more prone to illness: stomach ulcers, high blood pressure, and various addictions. Your breast cancer, although stressful, is not hopeless, and you should have a plan that will allow you to survive.

Some women with a new breast cancer diagnosis are able to look at their stressful life situations and make significant changes—switch to a less stressful job or career, end a difficult relationship, or restructure a financial burden, for example. These are usually good things to do and free up energy to address the important task at hand. While I don't want to discourage anyone from making important and healthy changes, we must remember that stress did not cause your cancer. A diagnosis of cancer can be a great motivator and a change agent, but I do not believe that women have caused their breast cancer by being overstressed, and we certainly encourage women to seek supportive networks or professional help when needed.

Alcohol

A fair number of epidemiologic studies have explored the link between alcohol and breast cancer. There is moderate evidence to suggest that there may be a connection between alcohol consumption, breast cancer incidence, and the risk of recurrence. If you search the Internet for *breast cancer and alcohol*, you will find millions of references. The data, however, is conflicting and difficult to interpret and for the most part rely on *retrospective studies*. If you choose to drink alcohol, it should be consumed in moderation (no more than three to five six-ounce glasses of beer or wine per week). In my opinion, the Life After Cancer Epidemiology (LACE) study, conducted by Kaiser Permanente in Northern California, is one of the best to date.

The study results seem to indicate that there was an increased risk of breast cancer recurrence in women who drank more than six ounces of alcohol per day. However, when results were more closely examined, it was only *postmenopausal obese women* who were at increased risk. Premenopausal and postmenopausal women with BMI less than 25 had no increase in risk. I interpret this to mean that moderate alcohol consumption is *not a major risk factor* for breast cancer, and it may not be a risk factor at all. The culprit may well be obesity, as we previously discussed.

Financial Concerns and Health Insurance

Earlier in this chapter, we discussed stress in relation to breast cancer. I cannot imagine anything more stressful than receiving a diagnosis of breast cancer and not being confident that one has reliable access to care and treatment. In the wealthiest nation in the world, this should not be an issue, but it is. For the increasing percentage of women without health insurance, gaining access to breast cancer treatment is a daunting task. Many states have programs for uninsured women with newly diagnosed breast cancer, and hopefully a local health care facility that can direct them to treatment.

There are resources available—comprehensive cancer centers, university teaching hospitals, and local community hospitals that have both teaching and research programs involved in the diagnosis and treatment of breast cancer. These institutions also have social workers or other health advocates available in addition to programs for women without financial resources. The Resources section of this book provides websites and contact information that can help in this regard.

Many women are eligible for research protocols that are supported by the government (National Cancer Institute) and the pharmaceutical industry. There are large and small foundations that help women in need. Most pharmaceutical companies have assistance programs to help women who are uninsured or underinsured. Even for women with health insurance, there are financial concerns and issues. Being able to work and support oneself during treatment is a common worry. Whether insurance will cover the treatment needed is another. Once you connect to a treatment center, these issues can be addressed with the help of the staff. No woman in this country should go without proper treatment.

The resources are available; the challenge is finding the connections.

Maintaining and Updating Your Medical Records

In this manual we recommend that you become educated and actively participate in your breast cancer care. We thus encourage you to maintain a copy of your medical records from initial diagnosis through treatment to follow-up care. This can be simply accomplished by gathering paper copies of your documents into a large three-ring notebook that has been divided into tabbed sections.

Alternatively, you can subscribe to a Web-based system that allows you to enter and access your health records. It makes sense to begin collecting your medical records right from the start, rather than trying to do so later when it becomes more difficult to retrieve records, reports, and images. We believe this is critically important in an evolving medical system. Whether you use this electronic format or you create your own, keeping track of your breast cancer medical history will help you stay informed and allow you to be more connected to your breast cancer journey.

Advocacy and Stewardship

❧ One of the brightest and most heartening things I have observed in my career as a breast oncologist has been the connections, support, and philanthropy that occur among women with breast cancer. This benevolent movement has generated major organizations and numerous support groups. The *sisterhood* with its pink ribbon logo is everywhere. Surely you will receive some benefit from this movement—perhaps from joining a support group, becoming a volunteer at your treatment center, or enrolling in research funded by a breast cancer walk or run. In my experience women deal with this illness in different ways.

The current task at hand is for you to get optimal treatment that will give you the best chance for a cure. Once you complete the "acute" treatment phase and become a *survivor*, you may want to become involved in some way in the breast cancer movement. My advice to patients is to *feel no pressure* to get involved; you should do so only when or if you are ready. Remember, there will be plenty of opportunities to join or volunteer. You are going to be a survivor for the rest of your life.

15

⁙

Conclusion

In this manual we have attempted to give you a foundation to launch you on your journey to a breast cancer cure. We have presented a large amount of new information that has become available since the previous edition was published. The new classification of breast cancer, based on genomic differences in cancer cells, is particularly relevant because it leads to markedly different treatment decisions.

Our understanding of breast cancer is expanding extremely rapidly. The information in this book will be current for a very short period as we continue to unravel the cancer cell's DNA. New, "targeted" agents will be developed based on new research and will be added to the dozen targeted drugs currently in use or being tested in early-stage breast cancer. At the time of the previous edition, there were only a few targeted drugs.

We hope new research will ultimately lead to the discovery of the causes of breast cancer, causes that have been elusive to researchers until now.

We discussed the importance of becoming involved in understanding your choices and the benefits of getting a second opinion. Second opinions become even more important as new techniques and treatments move rapidly from research into clinical practice.

Breast cancer is scary. Much of this fear stems from our inability to predict absolute outcomes in spite of our analysis with computers and genomic tests. Decisions may involve taking *risks* that must be weighed against *benefit*. Perhaps our most important task is to help you understand the risks and benefits of decisions that we are asking you to make.

It may be hard for you to believe, but you will get through this. In spite of the fear and uncertainty, the pain and discomfort, a diagnosis of breast cancer can have a "silver lining." Like other existential crises, it has the ability to help one refocus on what is important, what is sacred, and what is joyful. Breast cancer will force you to make decisions involving risk (there is no escape by default). You have the opportunity *to be afraid*, to be heroic, to take risks, and most important, *to survive*.

Anna Quindlen, in her wonderful little book *A Short Guide to a Happy Life*, describes her journey of transformation after her mother's illness.

> I learned to love the journey, not the destination. I learned that this is not a dress rehearsal, and that today is the only guarantee you get. I learned to look at all the good in the world and to try to give some back, because I believed in it completely and utterly. And I tried to do that, in part, by telling others what I had learned . . . By telling them this: Consider the lilies of the field. Look at the fuzz on a baby's ear. Read in the backyard with the sun on your face. Learn to be happy. And think of life as a terminal illness, because if you do, you will live it with joy and passion as it ought to be lived.

We hope that this survival manual will aid you on this "unchosen journey" of breast cancer and will help you to live long, be happy, and survive well.

Resources

The Internet can be a great source of information about breast health and breast cancer. Every day more and more information becomes available and in a very few minutes you can learn about the latest developments in breast cancer screening or research, locate a clinical research trial, or confirm that a surgeon is board certified. But how can you be sure that the information on a website is accurate and safe? Obtaining a referral from a trusted source is a good way to ensure that you are getting up-to-date information. You can also rely on well-known and trusted sites such as the National Cancer Institute (www.cancer.gov), the American Cancer Society (www.cancer.org), and even large university websites. To help you get started, we have included a number of trusted resources below that we believe can provide you with a wealth of information, education, and support.

Nonprofit Health Organizations

American Cancer Society (ACS)
www.cancer.org
The American Cancer Society is a nationwide, community-based, voluntary health organization dedicated to eliminating cancer as a major health problem by preventing cancer, saving lives, and diminishing suffering from cancer, through research, education, advocacy, and service. Email or call their helpline for cancer-related questions and for links to other resources.

American Institute for Cancer Research (AICR)

www.aicr.org

AICR offers a variety of services, from a Nutrition Hotline and healthy recipes to a special children's newsletter, all to help you eat and live more healthfully.

American Society of Clinical Oncology (ASCO)

www.cancer.net

The American Society of Clinical Oncology (ASCO) is the voice of the world's cancer physicians. ASCO's patient information website brings the expertise and resources of ASCO to people living with cancer and to those who care for and about them.

Breastcancer.org

www.breastcancer.org

Breastcancer.org is a nonprofit organization dedicated to providing the most reliable, complete, and up-to-date information about breast cancer. Its mission is to help women and families make sense of complex medical and personal information about breast cancer, so they can make the best decisions for their lives. On this site you will find reliable health information available for those affected by breast cancer and concerned about breast health.

Breast Cancer Care and Research Fund

www.breastcancercare.org

The Breast Cancer Care and Research Fund is a nonprofit organization that provides information and education to make breast cancer patients, their supporters, and the lay public more knowledgeable about breast cancer, treatments, and research.

Cancer Care, Inc.

www.cancercare.org

CancerCare, Inc., helps individuals and families cope with and manage the emotional and practical challenges resulting from cancer. Services for patients, survivors, loved ones, caregivers, and the bereaved include counseling and support groups, educational publications and workshops, and financial assistance. Professional oncology social workers provide assistance free of charge.

Cancer Support Community

www.cancersupportcommunity.org

The mission of the Cancer Support Community (CSC) is to ensure that all people impacted by cancer are empowered by knowledge, strengthened by action, and sustained by community. The CSC is an international nonprofit dedicated to providing support, education, and hope to people affected by cancer. This large global network of psychosocial oncology mental health professionals brings the highest quality cancer support to the millions of people touched by cancer. Support services are available through professionally led, community-based centers, in hospitals, at community oncology practices, and online, so that no one has to face cancer alone.

Kids Konnected
www.kidskonnected.org
This nonprofit provides education, understanding, and support for children who have a parent with cancer or who have lost a parent to cancer. The Kids Konnected website provides access to a 24-hour hotline, youth leadership, camps, and social events.

Living Beyond Breast Cancer
www.lbbc.org
Living Beyond Breast Cancer (LBBC) is a national education and support organization whose goal is to improve the quality of life for breast cancer patients and to encourage patients to take an active role in ongoing recovery or management of the disease regardless of educational background, social support, or financial means. LBCC offers programs and services to women affected by breast cancer, caregivers, and health care providers. They offer specialized programs and services for newly diagnosed patients, young women, women with advanced breast cancer, women at high risk for developing the disease, and African American and Latina women. Programs are available for caregivers and health care professionals to help better meet the needs of women affected by breast cancer.

National Breast Cancer Coalition
www.stopbreastcancer2020.org
The mission of the National Breast Cancer Coalition (NBCC) is to eradicate breast cancer. The NBCC encourages all those concerned about the disease to become advocates for action and change. The coalition informs, trains, and directs patients and others in effective advocacy efforts. Nationwide, women and men are increasing the awareness of breast cancer public policy by participating in legislative, scientific, and regulatory decisions, promoting positive media coverage, and actively working to raise public awareness. In 2010, NBCC launched a bold initiative, *Breast Cancer Deadline 2020*, a call to action for policy-makers, researchers, breast cancer advocates, and other stakeholders to end the disease by 2020.

National Cancer Center Network (NCCN)
www.nccn.org
NCCN and the NCCN Foundation® offer NCCN Guidelines for Patients® and corresponding NCCN Quick Guides™ for a variety of cancer types, treatment symptoms, and supportive care issues.

National Lymphedema Network
www.lymphnet.org
This international nonprofit group provides referrals, education, and guidance to lymphedema patients, health care professionals, and the general public. The National Lymphedema Network publishes a quarterly newsletter and holds a biennial conference for health care professionals.

National Patient Advocate Foundation
www.npaf.org
The National Patient Advocate Foundation (NPAF) is a national nonprofit organization that gives patients a voice in improving access to and reimbursement for high-quality health care through regulatory and legislative reform at the state and federal levels. NPAF translates the experience of millions of patients who have been helped by our companion, Patient Advocate Foundation, which provides professional case management services to individuals facing barriers to health care access for chronic and disabling diseases, medical debt crisis, and employment-related issues at no cost.

SHARE
www.sharecancersupport.org
The mission of SHARE is to create and sustain a supportive network and community of women affected by breast or ovarian cancer. SHARE brings women and their families and friends together with others who have experienced breast or ovarian cancer and provides participants with the opportunity to receive and exchange information, support, strength, and hope. SHARE's work focuses on empowerment, education, and advocacy to bring about better health care, an improved quality of life, and a cure for these diseases.

Susan G. Komen for the Cure
www.komen.org
Susan G. Komen for the Cure is the world's largest grassroots network of breast cancer survivors and activists. It is fighting to save lives, empower people, ensure quality care for all, and energize the scientific community to find the cure.

Its website provides education to help understand breast cancer, as well as information about research and research trials, numerous ways to get involved, and links to many other valuable breast cancer resources.

Y-Me National Breast Cancer Organization
www.y-me.org
Y-Me is a national nonprofit founded in 1978 with the mission to ensure, through information, empowerment, and peer support, that no one faces breast cancer alone. Peer support is the cornerstone of the Y-Me Breast Cancer Organization and peer counselors are available around the clock, 365 days a year.

Young Survival Coalition
www.youngsurvival.org
The Young Survival Coalition (YSC) is an international organization dedicated to the critical issues unique to young women diagnosed with breast cancer. YSC offers resources, connections, and outreach so women feel supported, empowered, and hopeful.

American Society of Plastic and Reconstructive Surgeons (ASPS)
www.plasticsurgery.org
The American Society of Plastic and Reconstructive Surgeons publishes numerous informational brochures and maintains this website to provide public education about plastic surgery. This site includes news on the latest advances and techniques in plastic and reconstructive surgeries and details about specific surgical procedures, including how to prepare for surgery, the types of anesthesia used, and how long recovery takes. Look for answers to the most frequently asked questions about plastic surgery and relevant statistics.

Academy of Nutrition and Dietetics
www.eatright.org
The Academy of Nutrition and Dietetics (AND) is the world's largest organization of food and nutrition professionals. ADA is committed to improving the nation's health and advancing the profession of dietetics through research, education, and advocacy. On the AND website you will find the latest food and nutrition information, hot topics in the field, nutritional guidance for different stages of life, and disease management and prevention tips, plus food safety guidelines and links to other resources. The AND website can also assist in locating a registered dietitian where you live.

Breastlink Medical Group
www.breastlink.com
Breastlink Medical Group is dedicated to delivering optimal care for women with breast cancer. The Optimal Care program is delivered through a team-based approach that includes radiologists, oncologists, surgeons, and pathologists focused specifically on the diagnosis, care, and treatment of breast cancer. Breastlink offers a comprehensive second-opinion service based on the team approach. To request a second opinion, please visit our website. There you will find complete instructions on how to obtain a timely, comprehensive opinion from our Optimal Care Breast Center.

National Society of Genetic Counselors
www.nsgc.org
The National Society of Genetic Counselors is an association of professionals who help people understand and adapt to the medical, psychological, and familial implications of genetic contributions to disease. This process includes: (1) Interpretation of family and medical histories to assess the chance of disease occurrence or recurrence, (2) Education about inheritance, testing, management, prevention, resources, and research, and (3) Counseling to promote informed choices and adaptation to the risk or condition. In addition to providing education, this website can assist in locating a genetic counselor in your area. (For an additional resource please see *My Family Health Portrait* under Government Agencies below.)

Government Agencies and Clinical Trials

ClinicalTrials.gov
www.clinicaltrials.gov
The National Institutes of Health (NIH), in collaboration with the Food and Drug Administration (FDA), has developed ClinicalTrials.gov to provide up-to-date information for locating federally and privately supported clinical trials for a wide range of diseases and conditions. ClinicalTrials.gov currently contains more than 100,000 research trials sponsored by the NIH, other federal agencies, and private industry. This website provides a wealth of information about cancer research and can help you to understand how clinical trials work, and the potential risks and benefits. The site presents research results and includes links to other agencies and resources, including a guide to understanding genetic conditions and the U.S. National Library of Medicine.

My Family Health Portrait
https://familyhistory.hhs.gov
My Family Health Portrait was developed in collaboration between the Office of the Surgeon General and the National Human Genome Research Institute. This Web-based tool helps users organize family health history information to give to their health care provider. Users can also save their family history information to their own computer and share with other family members. The tool is free to all users. No user information is saved on any computer of the U.S. government. After entering family history information, the Family Health Portrait tool will create and print out a graphical representation of your family's generations and the health disorders that may have moved from one generation to the next. That is a powerful tool for predicting diseases for which you may be at risk. Your health care provider can help you make use of this information. If you prefer to use a paper version of the tool to write in your family information, printable PDFs are available in several languages.

Office of Cancer Complementary and Alternative Medicine
www.cancer.gov/cam
The Office of Cancer Complementary and Alternative Medicine (OCCAM) was established to improve the quality of care for cancer patients, as well as those at risk for cancer and those recovering from cancer treatment, by contributing to the advancement of evidence-based complementary and alternative medicine (CAM) and the sciences that support it. This government office encourages collaboration between cancer researchers and CAM practitioners through lectures, conferences, and workshops. The office also identifies gaps in existing cancer CAM research and creates funding opportunities to increase the number of high-quality studies on this topic, as well as providing an expert review of CAM contents on behalf of NCI for institute-supported projects and programs.

National Cancer Institute
www.cancer.gov
The National Cancer Institute (NCI) is part of the National Institutes of Health (NIH) and is the federal government's principal agency for cancer research and training. The NCI conducts and supports research, training, health information dissemination, and other programs with respect to the cause, diagnosis, prevention, and treatment of cancer, rehabilitation from cancer, and the continuing care of cancer patients and their families. The NCI website provides information about all types of cancer, clinical trials research, cancer statistics, research funding, and publications of research results, among many other topics. A large number of valuable links are available on the NCI website. The Office of Cancer

Centers, a division of the NCI, is responsible for designating 66 nationwide Comprehensive Cancer Centers that are characterized by strong organizational capabilities, institutional commitment, and trans-disciplinary, cancer-focused science. These centers have experienced scientific and administrative leadership and state of the art cancer research and patient care facilities. A list of Comprehensive Cancer Centers can be found on this website.

U.S. Food and Drug Administration
www.fda.gov
The U.S. Food and Drug Administration (FDA) is an agency within the Department of Health and Human Services that is responsible for protecting the public health by assuring the safety, efficacy, and security of drugs, biological products, medical devices, our nation's food supply, cosmetics, and products that emit radiation, and by regulating the manufacture, marketing, and distribution of tobacco products. The FDA advances public health by speeding innovations that make medicines and foods safer, more effective, and more affordable and by providing the public with accurate, science-based information on medicines, foods, and tobacco use.

Diagnostic Company Resources—For Profit

Agendia
www.agendia.com
Agendia has developed a gene signature assay known as Blue Print that separates breast cancer into three types: (1) luminal, (2) basal, and (3) HER2. In addition, they have developed an RT-PCR assay known as Target Print that determines estrogen, progesterone, and HER2-positivity. Agendia has also developed a molecular diagnostic test called MammaPrint that can help predict the risk of breast cancer recurrence in the first five years after diagnosis. MammaPrint gives physicians a tool to help separate "high" risk from "low" risk early-stage breast cancer patients and better gauge "high" risk patients' need for chemotherapy.

Biotheranostics
www.biotheranostics.com
Biotheranostics is a commercial diagnostic laboratory that has developed a seven gene assay to predict the risk of systemic breast cancer recurrence at 0–10 years and 5–10 years. Two of the genes can assess the likelihood of responding to hormonal therapy.

Caris Life Sciences
www.carislifesciences.com
Caris Life Sciences has developed a test to examine the genetic and molecular makeup that is unique to each patient's tumor. By comparing the tumor's information with data from clinical studies from thousands of the world's leading cancer researchers, Caris can help the physician determine which treatments are likely to be most effective and which treatments are likely to be ineffective for each patient.

Genomic Health
www.genomichealth.com
Genomic Health is a molecular diagnostics company that is committed to improving the quality of cancer treatment through the development of genomic-based testing. The diagnostic tests, Oncotype DX breast cancer assay and Oncotype DX colon cancer assay, generate information that health care providers and patients can use in making decisions about treatment options. The Oncotype DX breast cancer assay is a test that examines a patient's tumor tissue and gives information about a particular patient's disease that can help individualize breast cancer treatment planning and identify options. Learn more about the Oncotype DX breast cancer assay on the Genomic Health website above or at www.oncotypeDX.com.

Myriad Genetics, Inc.
www.myriad.com
Myriad Genetics is a molecular diagnostic company that has developed tests to help identify genetic variations that are the most common causes of inherited cancers. These tests assist doctors and patients to understand the genetic basis of human disease and the role that genes play in the onset, progression, and treatment of disease. The Myriad Genetics website includes an online family cancer history tool and a hereditary cancer quiz that can help patients to evaluate their hereditary cancer risk.

Rational Therapeutics Cancer Laboratories
www.rational-t.com
Rational Therapeutics uses a patient's tumor tissue to test against a number of standard chemotherapies, and where possible, the newest targeted agents. Typically, the laboratory uses living tumor cells collected during biopsy or surgery and analyzes the response to individual drugs or a combination of drugs.

Glossary

Abraxane: Albumin-covered paclitaxel (Taxol).

acute: Sharp, intense, and of short duration.

adjuvant: Auxiliary, an aid to remove or prevent disease.

amino acids: The building blocks of proteins and the end products of protein digestion.

ancillary: Additional, auxiliary.

angiogenesis: Development of blood vessels.

areola: A circular pigmented area around the breast nipple.

assay: Analysis of a substance.

atypical lobular hyperplasia: Abnormally shaped cells proliferating excessively in the normal tissue arrangement of a breast lobule. Also called lobular neoplasia, type I.

autosomal dominant gene: Non-sex-based gene that requires only one copy in order to be expressed.

autosomal recessive gene: Non-sex-based gene that requires two copies in order to be expressed.

axillary lymph nodes: Lymph nodes in the armpit.

basal-type: A breast cancer type in the new classification based on genetic analysis. Also called triple-negative.

basement membrane: The separating membrane that provides a boundary from adjacent tissue.

biopsy: Excision of a small piece of living tissue for microscopic examination; usually performed to establish a diagnosis.

BRCA1: First discovered hereditary breast cancer gene mutation.

BRCA2: Second discovered hereditary breast cancer gene mutation.

chronic: Of long duration.

clear margin: Surrounding area of tissue that is clear of cancer cells after surgery.

colloid cancer: A rare ductal cancer also known as mucinous cancer.

combination chemotherapy: Combining drugs together in a single treatment.

cribriform: A pattern of cancer cell growth inside the breast duct that resembles mesh.

cystosarcoma phyllodes: A tumor of the breast that is of nonepithelial origin.

cytotoxic agents: Chemicals that destroy cells or prevent their multiplication.

differentiation: Cancer cells can be well, moderately, or poorly differentiated. The degree of differentiation describes how closely the cancer cell remains in appearance to a normal healthy cell. Well-differentiated cancer cells most closely resemble a normal cell, while poorly differentiated cells look least like normal cells and are therefore more malignant.

disease: The lack (*dis*) of ease; a pathological condition of the body.

DNA repair gene: A gene responsible for repairing DNA. A mutation in a DNA repair gene can lead to cancer. PARP is one example of a DNA repair gene.

dose dense: Intensifying the administration of chemotherapy by shortening the time interval between treatments.

ductal cancer in situ (DCIS): A cancer encapsulated within the breast ducts.

ductal cell: A cell from the duct of the breast.

electron beam boost: Use of radioactive particles to target a specific area of the body with additional radiation treatments.

enzyme: An organic catalyst produced by living cells but capable of acting independently. Enzymes produce chemical changes without being changed themselves.

epithelium: Cells that form a barrier to underlying tissue such as skin, ducts, and glands.

estrogen: The female sex hormone produced by the ovary. Estrogens are responsible for the development of secondary sexual characteristics and for cyclic changes in the vaginal epithelium and endothelium of the uterus.

excision: Surgical removal by cutting.

excisional biopsy: A biopsy in which an entire lesion is removed.

expander: A polyurethane flexible implant that is placed under the tissue and is enlarged manually by inserting a fluid, usually saline.

first-generation prognostic factors: Simple validated measures for predicting outcomes that have proved their usefulness in the past.

free radicals: Damage to tissue by molecules containing an odd number of electrons.

genistein: A phytoestrogen produced by soy products.

HER2 oncogene: An oncogene that is abnormally stimulated to produce an excess of protein, affecting cell division in the breast.

Herceptin: The brand name for trastuzumab, a drug that is used in HER2-positive breast cancer.

heterogeneous disease: A disease that does not manifest itself in the same way in every patient; having varying or dissimilar characteristics.

high-grade cancer: A cancer with a modified Bloom Richardson (BR) Grading Scale of 8 to 9, commonly with a high vascular component.

histologic grade: The microscopic measure and evaluation of the structure of a cancer.

homogeneous: Uniform in nature; a similar cause.

hormone: A substance that originates in a gland and is conveyed through the blood to another part of the body, stimulating it by chemical action to increase functional activity or increase secretion of other hormones.

hyperplasia: An increase in the number of cells in the lining of a gland.

hypothesis: An educated guess; a preliminary assumption based on enough observation to place it beyond mere speculation but requiring further experiments for verification.

infiltrating lobular carcinoma: Cancerous cells in the breast lobule that have spread through the basement membrane into the surrounding breast tissue.

in situ: In the normal place without disturbing the surrounding tissue, localized.

intraoperative radiation therapy (IORT): A form of breast irradiation administered as a single treatment during surgery.

invasive cancer: Cancer cells that penetrate the basement membrane, resulting in spread to healthy tissue.

isoflavone: A chemical found in soy products.

lobular carcinoma in situ (LCIS): A change in the breast lobule that increases the risk of breast cancer. It is a marker for breast cancer. The new nomenclature is lobular neoplasia, type 2.

lobular cell: A cell in the lobule of the breast; used for making milk.

lobular neoplasia: An abnormal accumulation of cells in the terminal lobule. When present, increases the risk of future breast cancer. Previously called LCIS.

local control: The control of cancer in the breast.

local recurrence: The return of cancerous cells to the breast.

luminal type: A type of breast cancer cell in the new breast cancer classification based on genetic analysis.

lumpectomy: Surgical removal of a tumor from the breast to clear margins not including the lymph nodes. Also known as a wide local excision.

lymphedema: Edema or swelling caused by obstruction of lymph channels.

lymph node: A rounded body consisting of an accumulation of lymphatic tissue found at intervals in the course of lymphatic vessels. Lymph nodes vary in size from a pinhead to an olive and can occur singularly or in groups. They produce lymphocytes and monocytes, and serve to filter matter from entering the bloodstream.

macroscopic: Visible to the naked eye; gross observation.

main tumor: A spontaneous new growth of tissue made up of abnormally dividing cells that form a mass.

markers: Tumor antigens that can be measured by blood tests.

mastectomy: See simple mastectomy; skin-sparing mastectomy.

mastitis: Inflammation or infection of the breast.

MBR scale: Modified Bloom-Richardson grading of the degree of malignancy.

metastatic disease: Movement of cancer cells from one part of the body to another.

microinvasion: Invasion of cancer cells through the breast duct into adjacent tissue at a microscopic level.

mitosis: The reproduction of cells; the process of cell division.

mitotic rate: Rate or speed of cell division.

mutation: Any basic alteration in form, quality, or some other characteristic. A change in genetic material of a chromosome that produces a new individual unlike its parents.

necrosis: Death of areas of tissue surrounded by healthy tissue.

neoadjuvant chemotherapy: The use of chemotherapy prior to curative surgery for local control.

neuropathy: Disease or damage of the nerves, causing lack of sensitivity or numbness.

oncogene: A gene that has the ability to induce a cell to become malignant. In addition to genes that induce tumor formation, there are antioncogenes that suppress tumors.

oncoplastic: Use of plastic and reconstructive techniques combined with oncologic surgery.

palpable: Capable of being touched or felt.

papillary cancer: A type of ductal cancer in the breast.

pathology report: An evaluation performed by a physician who specializes in the diagnosis of structural and functional changes in tissue that result from disease processes.

pedicle: A stem of tissue containing blood vessels allowing for the movement of that tissue to another area of the body.

perimenopausal: Around menopause.

phytochemicals: Chemicals found in plants.

phytoestrogen: An estrogen-like substance produced by plants.

pilot studies: Research investigations that explore a particular drug, technique, or idea.

placebo: Inactive substance given to patients as medicine; also used in control studies of drugs.

polyunsaturated fats: Fats made up of long-chain carbon compounds with many carbon atoms joined by double or triple bonds.

premalignant: Before metastasis; cancerous growth (as in lobular neoplasia).

progesterone: A steroid hormone from the corpus luteum and placenta. It is responsible for changes in the endometrium in the second half of the menstrual cycle, development of the maternal placenta, and development of the mammary glands.

prognosis: Estimated chance of recovery from the disease or chance that the disease will recur.

proliferate: To grow or multiply by rapidly producing new cells; to increase or spread at a rapid rate.

prophylactic: Contributing to the prevention of infection or disease.

quadrant: One-quarter; the breast is divided into four quadrants: upper outer, upper inner, lower outer, and lower inner.

randomized clinical trial: An investigation of the effects of a drug administered to human subjects. The goal is to define the clinical efficiency and pharmacological effects (toxicity, side effects, interactions) of the substance. This is done by a random method of assigning subjects to experimental treatment or nontreatment groups.

receptor: A cell component that combines with a drug, hormone, or chemical mediator to alter the function of the cell.

reconstruction: The action of constructing again. In breast reconstruction, the surgically altered breast is returned to its approximate original state.

recurrence: Return of the cancer.

remission: The period when cancer appears to be inactive.

satellite nodules: Small structures attached to the larger tumor.

sensitivity: The ability to react to stimuli. The value of a diagnostic test; the procedure of clinical observation.

sentinel node: The first lymph node draining a malignant tumor.

sequential chemotherapy: Using drugs in a singular manner, in a set sequence.

SERDs: Selective estrogen receptor downregulators.

SERMs: Selective estrogen receptor modulators.

simple mastectomy: Removal of the entire breast, leaving the adjacent lymph nodes and chest muscles intact. Also called a total mastectomy.

simulation: Radiation planning session designed to map out the radiation field.

skin-sparing mastectomy: A mastectomy that spares most of the skin overlying the removed breast tissue that can then be filled with tissue from a transfer or silicone or saline implant.

sporadic: Occurring occasionally or at scattered intervals.

stage: Denoting diagnosis and treatment on the basis of observation, pathology, and symptoms of patients.

staging system: The assessment of a cancer by size and quality.

state of the art: The best treatment available.

systemic control: The control of cancer throughout the body.

systemic spread: The spread of cancer cells to other organs via the bloodstream.

taxane: A class of chemotherapy drugs.

tissue transfer: Breast reconstruction by removing tissue from other parts of the body and replacing it in the breast.

toxicity: The extent or degree of being poisonous.

transverse rectus abdominis myocutaneous (TRAM) flap: Breast reconstruction surgery that uses tissue from the abdomen to rebuild the breast.

tubular cancer: A slow-growing, rare type of ductal cancer.

tumor: A growth of abnormal cells that forms a mass or lump. This can be benign or malignant.

tumor suppressor gene: A protective gene that normally limits the growth of tumors. When there is a mutation in a tumor suppressor gene it may fail to keep a cancer from growing. BRCA1 is an example of a tumor suppressor gene.

vascular system: The heart, blood vessels, lymphatics, and their parts considered collectively.

well-differentiated: Cancer cells that closely resemble the normal cells from which they developed.

wide local excision (WLE): See lumpectomy.

Index

Page numbers in *italics* refer to illustrations.

About the Author

DR. JOHN LINK is recognized as one of the world's leading breast cancer specialists. As the pioneer developer of Breastlink Medical Group, he established one of the first private, comprehensive breast care centers in the United States based on his innovative "optimal care" model that incorporates all aspects of screening, diagnosis, treatment, and follow-up within a single medical environment. Using this model, thousands of women from around the world have benefited from Dr. Link's philosophy that it is possible to provide women with individualized care tailored to their unique cancer situation using a team approach. By having all of the treating specialties together in one location, patients can feel confident that their treatment team is coordinated and working together to provide the very best care available.

Dr. Link was born in San Diego, California, and has spent his career practicing medicine in Southern California. He attended the University of Southern California (USC) for undergraduate studies, where he was an Academic All American. As a gifted runner and captain of the USC track team, Dr. Link held a world record in the two-mile relay (4×880). When his beloved track coach was diagnosed with cancer and died at the age of 42, Dr. Link knew that he wanted to pursue medicine and dedicate his career to the care and treatment of cancer patients.

While at the USC School of Medicine, he chose medical oncology as his focus and after graduation he decided to specialize exclusively in breast cancer. With the publication of this sixth edition of *The Breast Cancer Survival Manual*, Dr. Link continues to emphasize the importance of educating breast cancer patients about their disease and the different treatment options available so that they can be active participants in the development of their treatment plan. He believes all women should be empowered to survive this disease and that by understanding the risks and benefits of different treatment options, women will feel confident in the choices they make. Dr. Link's philosophy is that women should not only survive breast cancer, but they should survive well, and through careful evaluation and planning, women can receive optimal care for their unique situations.

In addition to his active medical practice, Dr. Link travels and lectures about breast cancer diagnosis and treatment to community groups, medical oncologists and other specialists, medical students, professional organizations, and private industry representatives. The first edition of the *Breast Cancer Survival Manual* was published in 1998, and since that time, Dr. Link has contributed to numerous other journal articles, poster sessions, and book chapters on breast cancer.

In 1995, Dr. Link founded Breastlink, a multispecialty breast cancer diagnostic and treatment medical group. The group included breast imaging, surgery, plastic surgery, medical oncology, breast cancer research, and patient supportive services. Breastlink became part of RADNET in 2008 and has grown to five centers in Southern California and a newly opened center in New York City.

Dr. Link and his wife, Nancy, have six children and live in Southern California, where they enjoy golf, travel, succulent gardening, and collecting contemporary art.